D1526949

EXPLORING
ADULT
SCOLIOSIS

A GUIDE TO TAKING BACK CONTROL
OVER YOUR SPINE AND YOUR LIFE

DR. TONY NALDA

Exploring Adult Scoliosis
A Guide to Taking Back Control over Your Spine and Your Life

ISBN 978-0-578-98451-3

CONTENTS

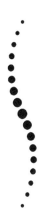

Introduction

BEING AN ADULT WITH scoliosis can be lonely, painful, and frustrating. I know this because I have worked with adults from all over the world who came to me with similar complaints.

Adults who have scoliosis experience lives marked by discomfort, and they are often told that there's nothing they can do about it, that is, until their condition becomes so severe that surgery becomes necessary.

If this sounds familiar to you, you might be wondering if there really is no other option than to watch and wait on your way to expensive, invasive surgery. I'm here to tell you that there is.

You don't have to just watch and wait as your condition progresses. Nor do you have to continue treating symptoms that only move around the body. You can treat your underlying structural condition, which is where all the pain and suffering comes from.

So, who am I, and why am I so passionate about this subject?

I was always drawn to a career in medicine, even when I was a kid. I felt drawn to the idea of helping other people. But I didn't always want to become a chiropractor, which is what I am today.

My dream was to become Tony Nalda, MD. However, my path was altered in my teenage years when I suffered terrible migraines.

I had enjoyed playing sports and participating in physical activities. Unfortunately, my migraines kept me from many of the things I loved during the sophomore and junior years of high school. I missed considerable time from school and experienced tremendous pain on an almost daily basis. In fact, I like to say that there was no such thing as a "good" day for me; the best I could hope for was a bad day instead of a *really* bad day. These migraines prevented me from living up to my potential. It was difficult to deal with, but luckily I had support from the right people.

Eventually, after living with my migraines for seven years between the ages of ten and seventeen, I saw a chiropractor. I was skeptical of what they could do to help me—I knew that there was a chance the treatments would have no impact on my migraines since they don't work the same on everyone—but I also knew that nothing else really worked for *me*. So I received a few treatments to start. Right away, I could tell that the treatments were helping me. The very first treatment was far from pleasant, but it gave me immediate relief. My pain was reduced through continued treatments, and the migraines disappeared after a while. I would never be the same at that point. No longer did I want to become Tony Nalda, MD; I wanted to become a chiropractor who could help people like my chiropractor helped me.

Chiropractic Is at the Center of a Scoliosis Treatment Revolution

In my adulthood, I became a general chiropractor, which allowed me to provide relief to many people. But there was something that nagged me about the way my scoliosis patients were responding to treatment. So I sought out ways in which chiropractic could be used to treat the condition.

In most cases of adult scoliosis, the condition and its treatment are managed by an orthopedic surgeon. What this means is that the goal of treatment is almost always viewed through the lens of surgery.

Surgeons are excellent at what they do. They receive extensive training and have undergone countless hours perfecting surgical techniques. The problem, to me, is that surgery is far from being the best approach to treating scoliosis.

When a surgeon leads the treatment approach, the operating table is practically inevitable for adults with scoliosis. Surgeons, given their specific training and experience, will almost always err on the side of surgical solutions versus more noninvasive, conservative treatments. Or they will attempt conservative treatment techniques, only to see them fail. Why? Because their specific training and worldview always come back to surgery being the ultimate gold standard for scoliosis treatment.

My belief in the effectiveness of chiropractic care had me questioning the status quo: Was surgery truly the best option for adults who wanted to relieve their scoliosis pain? Were there scoliosis-specific chiropractic techniques that could help patients build strength, flexibility, and mobility? Was it possible to help patients avoid surgery by engaging them in scoliosis-focused adjustments, therapies, and exercises?

My journey to becoming a scoliosis-focused chiropractor opened my eyes and made me see a whole new world of possibilities for adults who have the condition.

Today, I'm devoted to treating people who have scoliosis in a way that helps them build strength, function, and mobility. I help people avoid expensive and invasive surgeries. I also talk to other doctors about the benefits of scoliosis-focused chiropractic treatment.

My goal for this book is to inform, educate, and give you a little bit of hope as you decide what you should do next for your scoliosis. I have learned a great deal from treating patients of all ages over the years, and I'm dedicated to sharing my knowledge and wisdom so that patients can make better decisions regarding their care.

For adult patients, I believe this is of great importance. Adults who have scoliosis aren't given nearly as much attention as adolescents who have the condition. They are a forgotten segment of the population who deals with the condition, and for many adults, scoliosis gets worse and more painful every year. Usually, they are told there's nothing that can be done, other than surgery. I want to change that approach and that mindset. We can do better.

I will share insights and knowledge throughout this book designed to give you the facts about the condition you have. I'll debunk a lot of conventional wisdom and myths about the condition. Mostly, I aim to give you some hope. There is much you can do to live the life of your dreams. You don't need to be limited or defined by your condition. You can start a new life now.

Are you ready to begin?

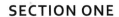

Do You Have Adult Scoliosis?

MAYBE YOU'VE ALREADY RECEIVED a diagnosis of adult scoliosis. Maybe you haven't, yet you suspect that the ailments and physical issues you've been experiencing are related to your spine.

Regardless, understanding adult scoliosis is important because the condition has the potential to create major changes in your life and the way you live it. If you do have adult scoliosis, it's critical to understand the nature of your condition and how it's a structural issue that cannot be treated effectively by addressing specific symptoms. If you haven't received a diagnosis but suspect that your spine and its curvature is the common denominator among your ailments and issues, learning the facts about the condition will help you make more intelligent, informed decisions about your future.

Scoliosis is a complex condition that impacts a large number of adults, even though it's seen by many as an adolescent issue. But what happens to all those teenagers when they grow up? The scoliosis doesn't disappear; it only progresses and becomes increasingly severe over time. Sometimes, scoliosis that was mild or undetectable in adolescence comes alive in adulthood, creating symptoms and difficulties that never existed before. Other times, adults develop scoliosis in adulthood due to the degeneration of their bodies from aging and other factors.

The truth is that the segment of the population with the highest percentage of scoliosis cases is adults, not adolescents. In fact, the percentage of cases increases over time as people age (*see graphic*).

What is the most common age with people with scoliosis?

• 1% to 5% in children

• 4%-10% above the age of 18 years

• 9% in over 40 year olds

• 30%+ in over 60 year olds

• 50%+ in over 90 year olds

The prevalence of Scoliosis increases with age ....

2010 Journal of Bone and Joint Surgery - British Volume, Vol 92-B, Issue 7, 980-983 Spine 2011 Apr 20;36(9):731-6.

This book is all about helping you find hope. I am here to provide education and insight into your condition so you can make choices that put you in the best possible position to enjoy life and live it to its fullest. It is truly possible, even if your scoliosis has become severe and painful in adulthood. I have seen patients transform their lives completely—with no surgery. I can tell you how you can join them, too. But first, I think I should start by explaining what adult scoliosis is (and how there are two main types of the condition), how it differs from adolescent scoliosis, and how you can use your knowledge to make choices that serve you and your spine moving forward.

Let's get started.

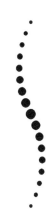

CHAPTER ONE

What Is Adult Scoliosis?

GETTING OLDER COMES WITH its share of perks and priv-ileges: You gain wisdom and perspective with age. If you're a parent, you've had the chance to watch your children grow, learn, and become adults you can be proud of. In your professional life, you have probably risen through the ranks to a place of relative comfort and stability. You've experienced success, which means you should be feeling better than you've ever felt, right?

Unfortunately, that might not be your reality, even if you feel you've done everything to keep your body healthy, flexible, and pain-free.

Many of us have placed a priority on health and fitness in our adult lives, which can provide a renewed sense of youthfulness and vitality. If you're like many of your peers, you've incorporated a fitness routine into your schedule, and that's a great thing. I know many people over the age of forty who say they're in the best shape of their lives—and they have the bodies to prove it. Adulthood can be a time of rebirth and rejuvenation for the human body.

Sadly, adulthood is also the time in our lives when the body begins to feel the effects of a life of usage and impact. For some, new conditions arise out of the continuous degeneration of the body. Others experience pain and additional symptoms related to accidents or injuries. There are also many adults who have had structural issues with their bodies their entire lives but are only now experiencing painful symptoms or negative effects on their ability to live life to the fullest. Those little, insignificant aches and pains that you tolerated in your youth are now demanding your full attention, getting in the way of your lifestyle.

What about you?

Do you find yourself experiencing pain or discomfort on a regular basis, but you're not sure why?

Have you noticed your posture becoming worse, or are you somehow getting "shorter"?

Have you noticed yourself "running out of gas" by the late afternoon or early evening because of pain that seems to come from the spine?

Are you experiencing asymmetrical joint pain, particularly in your lower extremities (knees, hips, and feet)?

Have you suspected that your spine could be the cause of your issues but have been told you're wrong?

You're at a point where you want answers, and you crave a roadmap to a fuller, more pain-free life. You have probably tried a number of promising remedies and modalities that just didn't work. All the strengthening, stretching, yoga, and exercise that have been recommended to you has not relieved your symptoms. You've done the work to heal yourself, and have exhausted nearly every possibility. Yet no one will validate what you feel to be the source of your pain and discomfort: your spine.

It's frustrating, isn't it?

In reality, most orthopedic surgeons will be reluctant to even mention that scoliosis is a potential source of a patient's concern. In my view, this is because they simply don't have the tools or techniques to treat the condition until it becomes surgical. In other words, they are highly unlikely to make diagnoses that they're unable to address with surgery. That's why they advise patients to watch and wait. Or they prescribe pain medications, which only serve to kick the can down the road a little further. They have no real treatment options to offer, so they continue to recommend additional delays and stopgap solutions. Of course, this approach leaves patients in pain and suffering as the underlying condition worsens.

I have numerous patients who have been shocked to learn that scoliosis has been evident in X-rays, films, and scans for quite a while; the condition was not revealed, however, by their previous providers. When I see such evidence, I have no problem letting people know about the realities of their condition. That's largely because I know how to treat it effectively. I can describe a treatment plan and what it's meant to address. I can be honest and forthcoming about what treatment will require and what patients can expect. Surgeons cannot provide this type of care because they are just not trained to do so. They're trained to perform surgeries.

If you've been frustrated by the narrow range of options available to you, or you suspect that your providers are giving you the runaround, it may be because you are seeking solutions from people who only have one option to offer. Yes, it's acknowledged to be the standard model of treatment, but it's far from being the most effective.

When I meet with adult patients in my practice at the Scoliosis Reduction Center, I hear many of the same stories about their journeys to me. They've tried everything. They're told by "experts" that the spine isn't the issue; it must be something else. So they go through years of their lives spending time, money, and energy chasing relief that never arrives. Eventually, they begin to listen to their bodies and their own intuition again. Intuitively, they have a sense that what they are experiencing is an underlying structural condition, and many of them are right about that. Then, finally, they become validated when they receive a diagnosis of adult scoliosis.

Scoliosis in adults isn't well understood by the general public, largely because it's seen as a condition that affects adolescents. Therefore, it may not have occurred to you that it was possible to develop the condition at your age. Or you might have ruled out the possibility of scoliosis because you were tested in your adolescence and no abnormal curvature was found.

The truth is that scoliosis is a condition that affects people of all ages. Yes, it tends to develop and become evident in adolescence, but that doesn't mean it can't arise in adults who have shown no previous evidence of the condition. Furthermore, it can go completely undetected in adolescence, presenting no negative issues until well into one's adulthood. This is because scoliosis is a progressive condition—it never improves or stabilizes on its own. So if you had a very minor, unacknowledged curvature in your adolescence, it probably didn't present any challenges. But without intervention, that curve has only grown more dramatically abnormal over the years. Many cases of scoliosis are just like this—adolescent idiopathic scoliosis exists in a patient's youth but progresses so slowly that it doesn't become problematic until well into adulthood.

I like to think of it as a turtle-and-the-hare scenario. Scoliosis in adolescents often progresses rapidly, like the hare. It makes itself obvious, even to the naked eye. On the other hand, adult scoliosis operates like the turtle—slow and steady. It doesn't work rapidly, so people tend to ignore it, or they fail to take it seriously. Eventually, as in the classic fable, the turtle catches up. But it doesn't just catch up; it *becomes* the rabbit.

Another way to picture it is like this: Developing adult scoliosis is like gaining a half pound each year. It's not noticeable. It doesn't affect your life or force you to make changes, that is, until several years go by and you realize how much your body has changed.

In adults, when curvatures progress, they cause a great deal of pain and discomfort, which is typically not the case for adolescents with the condition. Because adolescents have young, growing bodies, they don't experience the effects of compression and pressure on the spine that adults endure. For young people, growth and development in the teenage years can be awkward and emotionally challenging, but for those who have adolescent idiopathic scoliosis, the growth of the body actually provides relief from scoliosis.

For adults, pain is almost always a characteristic of their scoliosis. But because it manifests in so many different ways—and, potentially, in so many different areas of the body—its true source is often disguised. Over time, adults with scoliosis develop aches and pains. Then they and their health-care providers address the symptoms without investigating the underlying causes. The temporary relief provided by addressing the symptoms can be profound, and it can provide hope. But it's only ever just that—temporary. Without addressing the underlying structural causes of the symptoms, patients find themselves constantly chasing relief. They never catch up, though. Whether it's the turtle or the hare, scoliosis will always win the race unless the abnormal spinal curvature is addressed and reduced.

Adult scoliosis can be demoralizing in so many ways. It isn't as well publicized as adolescent idiopathic scoliosis. And it tends to go unrecognized by doctors and other health-care providers, even when patients suspect that the spine is the ultimate underlying source of the pain. It keeps people from living their fullest, healthiest lives. It makes people want to give up when they recognize that they are stuck in a cycle. First, there's pain and discomfort. Then there's the pain and discomfort of seeking relief. That's followed by a temporary easing of their pain when specific symptoms are addressed. Inevitably, the pain returns. And frustrations continue to grow as providers continue to do everything but address the underlying cause. Shockingly, it's fairly common for doctors to tell their patients that there's nothing that can be done, and that they must "learn to live with it."

Scoliosis, being a progressive condition, only allows for so many trips through this cycle. For many adults with scoliosis, this means that they engage in ineffective treatments up until the point when surgery becomes "necessary." And then it's too late to address the spine's abnormal curvature and reduce it.

This cycle doesn't have to be repeated.

I know this cycle must seem familiar to you. Otherwise, it's unlikely that you would have picked up this book. And you're probably worried that if you don't do something soon to address your spine's structural issues, you'll have no choice but to end up on the surgeon's operating table.

Perhaps you're experiencing pain and looking for validation that your spine is the source of your discomfort. You've sought treatment for all the symptoms; now you just want someone to tell you what you have suspected as the truth for some time.

Or maybe you've already received a diagnosis of adult scoliosis, and you are adamant about avoiding surgery. So now you're looking for solutions outside the world of mainstream orthopedic treatments. You don't want to limit your life and your options by engaging in invasive surgery. And you know there's a lot more to life than just getting through your days before pain takes over.

It's also possible that you've talked to someone who has avoided scoliosis surgery through alternative treatments. But the excitement is blunted by your orthopedic surgeon, who reiterates that such success is impossible. You want to believe that there are treatments that can help you avoid surgery, but you're skeptical. Who is right? What can you believe?

Regardless of why you are here, I want you to know that there is hope for people like you. Surgery isn't the only way forward. And it's possible to reduce—and even reverse—the abnormal spinal curvatures that are causing so much pain and hardship.

Before you move forward, though, I believe it is critical to understand adult scoliosis and why it impacts life the way it does. In many ways, it's similar to adolescent scoliosis. However, if you intend to treat it properly, you need to know how it is unique in adults such as yourself.

Of course, every case of adult scoliosis is its own unique entity. No two spines are alike. Therefore, an effective one-size-fits-all treatment for adult scoliosis will never exist. Treating scoliosis effectively also requires hard work and commitment from the patient. If you have the condition, it's important to know that stabilizing your spine or reducing your curvature cannot be done quickly, easily, or without effort. So beware of quick fixes or "magic pill" solutions, which are always backed by empty promises.

There's not a lot of advocacy for people who suffer from adult scoliosis. It isn't a hot topic in our media or culture by any means. And let's face it—the condition predominantly affects women over the age of forty, which is a demographic that often gets ignored. You may feel alone and unempowered to take action, but it doesn't have to be that way. With knowledge about scoliosis and hope for your future, you can find a way to reduce your curvature, reduce your pain, and increase your ability to live your best life.

As an adult with scoliosis, feeling validation and hope are incredibly important. Knowing what scoliosis can do to the adult body is crucial as well. Additionally, I believe it's helpful to understand the history of the condition, how it affects the body, and how people have been treating it across history.

Scoliosis has been a recognized medical condition for centuries. You've heard of the Hippocratic oath (i.e., "do no harm") that physicians take, right? That oath is named after the ancient Greek physician Hippocrates, who wrote about spinal deformities as far back as 460 BC. Centuries later, another Greek physician, Galen, identified and defined abnormal spinal curvatures, using specific terminology that we still utilize today.

In fact, terms like *lordosis*, *kyphosis*, and *scoliosis* were coined by Galen almost two thousand years ago.

Galen observed that spines are three-dimensional structures. This was an incredibly important innovation. I like to talk about scoliosis as a "3-D condition," and this is what I mean; the spine's curvature cannot be understood in two dimensions. For example, lordosis describes a backward-bending curve as viewed from the side. A normal spine features a certain amount of lordosis in the cervical and lumbar regions. Kyphosis describes a forward-bending curve as viewed from the side. Again, a normal, healthy spine will display a certain amount of kyphosis, but in the thoracic (midback) region. Scoliosis describes an abnormal curvature of the spine when viewing from the front or back.

In most cases of adult scoliosis, one or more side-to-side curves may exist. The result could be a C- or S-shaped spinal curvature, which may not be obvious to untrained observers. It may also be combined with abnormal kyphosis or lordosis curvatures, which should reinforce the need to view it as a "3-D condition." The way the condition impacts one adult could be considerably different from how it affects another as well. Again, no two cases of scoliosis are alike.

How Well Do You Know Scoliosis Terminology?

Scoliosis is one of the more complicated medical conditions a person can have. In reality, scoliosis is one word that describes any abnormal lateral or sideways curvature in a person's spine. There is typically much more going on than just a single abnormal curvature. With the complexity of the condition comes several complex terms. Here's a cheat sheet:

Kyphosis—When viewing the body from the side, kyphosis appears as a forward-bending curve. A normal spine features a natural amount of kyphosis in its thoracic region. But when a forward-bending curvature becomes excessive, it is referred to as *kyphotic*. Kyphosis is often found in combination with scoliosis. This is common among adults with De Novo scoliosis. When this is the case, the condition is technically known as *kyphoscoliosis*. This terminology is also used to describe cases when a normal *lordosis* has bent completely in the opposite direction. When this happens, it's known as *cervical kyphosis*.

Lordosis—When viewing the body from the side, a backward-bending curvature of the spine in the cervical or lumbar region is known as *lordosis*. It can be problematic whether it is excessively large or excessively small.

Dextroscoliosis—This is the term that is used to describe an abnormal curvature that goes to the right side of the body (*dextro*, in medical terminology, means "right"), usually in the thoracic region of the spine. This is the most commonly seen curvature among people who have scoliosis. Why? The body has a natural inclination to avoid the heart, which is located to the left of the torso's center. This type of curvature is seen on its own (forming a C-curve), but is also seen combined with other curvatures that go in the opposite direction (forming an S curve).

Levoscoliosis—This term describes an abnormal scoliosis curvature that goes to the left side of the body (*levo*, in medical terminology, means "left"). In typical cases, this type of curvature appears in the lumbar region of the spine. For those adults who have De Novo scoliosis, the condition tends to present itself with this type of lumbar curvature. Sometimes, levoscoliosis can appear in the thoracic region of the spine, in which case an MRI is typically recommended. That's because the presence of levoscoliosis in the thoracic region could be a sign that another condition (i.e., spinal cord tethering, spinal cord tumor, or Chiari syndrome) is actually acting as the underlying cause.

Why is it so complicated? Consider the fact that your spine is made up of twenty-four different, individual vertebrae. The vertebrae are grouped into three regions of the spine: Seven cervical vertebrae make up the neck region of the spine. The middle back is made up of twelve thoracic vertebrae. And the lower back consists of five lumbar vertebrae. Each region is different, and each vertebra can serve as a point of articulation. The many different ways in which a spine can bend, twist or curve abnormally is nearly infinite. What's more, countless factors figure into the manner in which scoliosis manifests in the body. This is why every case is unique. And it's why each case must be treated individually.

For adults who have the degenerative (De Novo) form of scoliosis, the abnormal curvature most likely exists within the lumbar region. However, it could also combine with scoliosis that exists in the other spinal regions. In many cases of adult scoliosis, the condition affects both the lumbar and thoracic regions of the spine. These curves are known as "double major curves."

Another factor to consider is that there are two major types of adult scoliosis. Adolescent idiopathic scoliosis in adults, which is also known as *ASA*, refers to scoliosis that has existed since childhood and progressed into the patient's adult years. Combined with the body's normal changes and deteriorations, this form of adult scoliosis typically puts the patient in the type of pain that urges them to seek treatment. Because this type of scoliosis is idiopathic, by definition, it has no known cause. Nevertheless, treatment should focus on the underlying structural issues that cause the condition and its symptoms.

The other major type of adult scoliosis is the aforementioned De Novo scoliosis. Also known as *degenerative scoliosis* (DS), this form of the condition usually appears only after the patient has reached middle age, well after the full development of their skeletal structures. In most cases, De Novo scoliosis is precipitated by the degeneration of the patient's spinal disks in an uneven manner. Those who have this type of scoliosis also frequently develop spinal stenosis, which is the abnormal narrowing of the spinal canal. As a result, a patient may experience a troubling amount of pain and stiffness as well as numbness or weakness in the limbs.

I will describe and investigate the two major forms of adult scoliosis in the next chapter.

Understanding adult scoliosis can be intimidating. But your knowledge and expertise will help you considerably as you advocate for yourself on your way to healing. Understanding your condition means recognizing that your case of scoliosis is completely unique; it can only be treated effectively by developing a plan specific for your needs and your body. I also believe that it's never too late to act and to seek treatments that address the underlying structural issues that contribute to your scoliosis.

With that in mind, I'd like to move forward by exploring the two major types of adult scoliosis: how they differ, how they are similar, and what you can do to seek the healing you require.

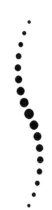

CHAPTER TWO

The Different Types of Adult Scoliosis

FOR ADULTS WITH SCOLIOSIS, pain is usually the defining characteristic of their condition. However, adolescents who have the condition tend to experience little to no pain. Why is that the case?

As I mentioned in the previous chapter, adolescent bodies provide a natural form of pain prevention from scoliosis. Scoliosis pain typically arises from the compression of the spine. Growing bodies are engaged in continuous upward movement that works to decompress the spine and keep pain from appearing. However, adult bodies that have stopped growing don't benefit from this natural relief from spinal compression.

Have you ever wondered why you can feel so good in the morning but by the late afternoon you want to call it a day? It's because your spine can only handle being upright for so long before it begins to compress, causing pain and discomfort. The pain, fatigue, and near-constant discomfort of scoliosis is the ultimate motivator for adults who have the condition. It is possible that they have had the condition since childhood. But because of the natural decompression that happens in adolescent bodies, they just didn't begin to feel it until well into adulthood.

I write about pain here because it's the common factor uniting the two major forms of adult scoliosis. If you've begun to experience pain that you suspect is caused by your spine, you may assume that what you have is a new condition—something that has only been with you in adulthood. While that may, in fact, be the case, it is possible that you've had scoliosis for much of your life. It just hasn't caused challenges until now. Here's the truth: If you're an adult with scoliosis and you're *not* experiencing pain, you are in the minority. It's really only a matter of time before pain shows up in your life.

The truth is that, by far, the most common form of adult scoliosis is adolescent idiopathic scoliosis in adults, or *ASA*. This is the type of scoliosis that has existed since childhood, and has progressed into adulthood. Remember the turtle-versus-hare scenario from the previous chapter? That's what I'm referring to here. In the case of ASA, the turtle is the one winning the race. In other words, the condition progressed so slowly, steadily, and subtly that detecting it was virtually impossible until adulthood. Either the patient was diagnosed with a mild form of scoliosis in childhood and was put on the path of watching and waiting, or they were never diagnosed at all.

In adults, the idiopathic scoliosis that has existed since adolescence progresses alongside the natural degenerative changes of aging. The spine deteriorates as its abnormal curvature progresses, creating a one-two punch of pain and discomfort that spurs the patient to seek a diagnosis—and relief. Spinal joints that are engaged in natural deterioration from age are put under additional stress from the continuously progressing scoliosis curvature. This is typically where the intense pain comes from.

Again, this is why you may feel so fresh, energized, and pain-free in the mornings, while at night, you simply run out of energy or must surrender to your pain.

Four Types of Idiopathic Scoliosis

Understanding scoliosis is a little easier when you can break it down into types. *Idiopathic* is one type of scoliosis, but it actually contains four different subtypes, broken down by age. These subtype definitions aren't perfect, by any means, but learning about them can help you understand how the condition can arise and progress through the years.

Infantile Idiopathic Scoliosis—This type of idiopathic scoliosis appears between birth and the age of three. It may surprise you to learn that children this young and undeveloped can have scoliosis, but it's true. In the vast majority of cases, this type of scoliosis has a small chance of resolving itself without treatment, with patients typically going on to live normal lives. However, when cases of this type fail to resolve on their own, they can present numerous challenges. Frequent checkups are necessary to observe and manage the condition. Additionally, children with this form of scoliosis are unable to engage in scoliosis-specific exercises or physical therapy that would benefit older patients. Therefore, they must be subject to aggressive, passive treatments that don't involve surgery. But surgery remains an option, even at this tender age. Methods for treating infantile scoliosis surgically involve inserting expandable rods into the body.

Juvenile Idiopathic Scoliosis—This type of idiopathic scoliosis is diagnosed when abnormal spinal curvatures appear in patients between the ages of three and ten. While this form of the condition isn't as common as adolescent idiopathic scoliosis, it accounts for approximately 10–15 percent of all cases, so it's significant.

Treatment options for this age group are more robust than those that are available in the infantile group, but great care must be taken to ensure that treatment is combined with caring support from teachers, parents, and other important people in the child's life. Children at this age can benefit from a scoliosis-specific therapy and exercise program, and the rate of success is quite high, but it's a tough road. That is why extra emotional support and coaching can be so crucial.

Adolescent Idiopathic Scoliosis—This is easily the most well-documented type of scoliosis that exists. It is also the most commonly diagnosed. Adolescent idiopathic scoliosis (AIS) is diagnosed in children between the ages of eleven and eighteen, and it makes up more than three-quarters of idiopathic scoliosis cases diagnosed in childhood. This age range coincides with the range during which children experience the greatest physical growth. The skeleton works hard to reach maturity during this stage of life, and if it's affected by scoliosis, that means it must be taken seriously to ensure that the body develops in a healthy manner. The risk of severe progression becomes higher in this age range as well. This is the ideal time to act, and it's a great time to motivate a teenager to take their treatment seriously. At this age, patients are concerned with their appearances and their futures. They don't want to let things like surgery get in the way of the fast track they're on, so I find that they are usually pretty eager to participate in treatments, physical therapy, and scoliosis-based exercise, regardless of how grueling they may be. Why? Because teenagers will do just about anything to avoid the extremely unappealing prospect of surgery.

Adolescent Idiopathic Scoliosis in an Adult—Once a patient has reached adulthood at the age of eighteen, a distinction is made: adolescent idiopathic scoliosis (AIS) becomes adolescent idiopathic scoliosis in an adult (ASA). This distinction is little more than a formality used to acknowledge that a patient is an adult and no longer a child. The underlying scoliosis doesn't change (apart from its normal, natural progression); the person with the scoliosis just reaches a new category of life. At this stage of life, however, the body has stopped growing, and the patient has reached skeletal maturity. As a result, pain management becomes a more pressing concern. However, it's still possible to treat the condition in a manner that not only reduces pain but also reduces the abnormal spinal curvature and slows its progression. This requires a treatment regimen that involves scoliosis-specific chiropractic care, physical therapy, exercise, and, potentially, bracing. In my experience, adults are motivated to do the work because it means that they'll experience less pain. Once the pain begins to subside, it boosts their motivation further, allowing them to take steps designed to restore function and ability as well.

Although the majority of scoliosis cases in adults are those that have existed since adolescence (ASA), there is another major category of the condition. De Novo scoliosis, which is also referred to as *degenerative scoliosis*, or DS, is the form of the condition that arises in adults in middle age (or older), whose skeletal structures have developed fully. This form of adult scoliosis is often referred to as *adult onset scoliosis*. Regardless of whether you're familiar with the terms *degenerative scoliosis*, *De Novo scoliosis*, or *adult onset scoliosis*, you should know that they're all describing the same condition.

De Novo scoliosis is a degenerative condition, which explains why it is commonly called *degenerative scoliosis*. *Degenerative*, in this case, refers to the degeneration of the body's spinal joints. The breakdown of these joints leads to an abnormal side-to-side curvature in the spine. Most cases of this type of scoliosis are diagnosed in adults at middle age or older, with the age range of thirty-five to sixty-five being the most prominent.

Most of the time, De Novo scoliosis appears in the lumbar spine. It produces a C-shaped curvature. By itself, this abnormal curvature can cause a great deal of pain. But that's not the full extent of what happens when a person develops scoliosis at this stage of life. The rest of the body—including internal organs— must compensate for the abnormal structuring of the spine. It's a chain reaction that can lead to a number of health problems, many of which are commonly treated without addressing the underlying condition of the spine. Therefore, many adults with scoliosis endure continuously increasing pain and discomfort, treating symptoms for months and even years before arriving at the root cause.

The wear and tear I described with regard to degenerative scoliosis can be caused by a condition known as *spondylosis*. It's a type of arthritis that occurs due to uncorrected asymmetrical alignment, causing disks and joints of the spine to deteriorate in a progressive fashion over time. Although it can be correlated with the progression of aging, it can arise in anyone who has experienced asymmetrical alignment in their spines. Consider a car that's out of alignment—parts and components on one side are likely to deteriorate faster than on the other. It may seem like a symptom of the vehicle getting older, but it has nothing to do with the car's age; it's all about the misalignment that has caused the deterioration. It is also not unusual for abnormal bone spurs to show up as well, which can contribute to even more abnormal twisting and slipping of the spine. Eventually, the curvature of the spine becomes so abnormal over time that it leads to scoliosis.

Consider that adults also must take on challenges associated with conditions like osteoporosis, compression fractures in the vertebrae, and the degeneration of spinal disks. All of these conditions cause a certain amount of pain and discomfort, which individuals compensate for by leaning one way or the other, or by twisting their bodies to relieve their strain. These types of compensations only serve to exacerbate the condition and cause scoliosis to potentially progress more rapidly.

By definition, those who have De Novo scoliosis developed the condition as adults. However, it's possible that many cases of degenerative scoliosis actually began in adolescence as idiopathic scoliosis. These cases were never diagnosed, though, because the condition didn't cause pain or limitations.

Detecting scoliosis as early as possible creates the best-case scenario for any patient. Unfortunately, early detection is quite challenging. Teenagers who have scoliosis typically don't experience pain from the condition. Therefore, they have no reason to voice concerns about their bodies to their parents or health-care providers. There is simply no opportunity for a diagnosis of scoliosis to be revealed because to teens, they are just going about their normal lives. Often, abnormal spinal curvatures caused by scoliosis in adolescence remain subtle or barely noticeable well into adulthood.

How Do You Know if You Have Scoliosis?

Many adults who have scoliosis were not diagnosed in adolescence, even though they may have had the condition since their teenage years or earlier. If you suspect you might be one of these people, you're probably wondering how you can tell, for sure, if you have the condition.

It is likely that you have experienced pain or other ailments for a while. You have been treating the symptoms, and yet, new symptoms seem to keep arising. You've also probably received a number of different diagnoses, all pertaining to your symptoms without addressing their underlying cause.

I meet countless adult patients with scoliosis who just want validation. They feel deep down that something more structural is going on in their bodies, causing the symptoms they've been experiencing. But their concerns seem to fall on deaf ears as they endure increasing amounts of pain, discomfort and exhaustion.

Thankfully, there are a few things you can do if you suspect you may have adult scoliosis and want to know for sure.

The fact is that it will be hard for you to tell if you have scoliosis on your own. You are with your body every day, and the slow, steady, gradual changes that take place in your spine are likely to go undetected by you. So it's possible that someone close to you has noticed something unusual about your body.

Of course, scoliosis is a progressive condition. Sooner or later, the abnormal curvature of your spine will advance to the point that you'll notice your clothes fitting oddly. Perhaps one pant seems shorter or longer than the other, or the fit of your blouse or shirt becomes misaligned and off-center. You may notice this yourself, or it may be pointed out to you by someone else.

Eventually, scoliosis becomes obvious and visible from behind. While the spine will present a natural curvature when viewed from the side, it should appear as a straight line, up and down, from the back. A side-to-side curvature, when viewed here, is the tell-tale sign that scoliosis is present.

Take a close look at your body. Does one hip appear to be higher than the other? Do your shoulders appear to be uneven? Does your head seem to be off-center in relationship to the rest of your body? These are all signs that scoliosis could be present.

A simple visit to the doctor can reveal quite a bit too. Many health-care providers will observe physical signs that could indicate the presence of scoliosis. As an adult, these signs will be more prominent, and may even be detected during a routine physical examination. If your provider suspects that you may have scoliosis, there are further noninvasive tests that may be done.

Perhaps you've heard of the *Adams forward bend test.* It is actually one of the most common tests designed to detect cases of scoliosis. With it, you and your health-care provider can make some useful observations. It's a simple test, but can be quite revealing without the benefit of X-rays or scans.

This test isn't foolproof. Scoliosis can exist, even if a person appears normal. Also, the Adams forward bend test is quite effective at detecting thoracic scoliosis. But it isn't as effective at detecting lumbar scoliosis. Ultimately, it is a reliable method for detecting some common scoliosis indicators. These can include uneven hips or shoulders or a visible curvature in the spine. If your provider uses a tool known as a *scoliometer,* they'll be able to measure your trunk rotation, which can be used to zero in on the curvature's location and size.

Ultimately, knowing whether you have scoliosis or not will depend on you. You'll have to be your own best advocate as you move forward. Fortunately, your knowledge of the condition will serve you well and allow you to ask good questions about the symptoms you're experiencing. As is the case with many adults who have scoliosis, you've probably suspected something was wrong with your spine for a while now. And if you're experiencing ever-increasing amounts of pain and discomfort, it's highly possible that the pain and discomfort is being caused by scoliosis, whether your abnormal curvature is obvious or not.

The Cobb Angle Explained

When we measure abnormal spinal curvatures, we use something called the *Cobb angle*. If you have been doing some scoliosis research, you've probably heard of this unusually named measurement and wondered where it came from. Was there an actual person named Cobb?

I will answer the last question first: Yes, Dr. John R. Cobb was an American orthopedic surgeon who first described his unique measurement technique back in 1948.

Basically, the Cobb angle is a measurement of the spine's curvature using degrees. Doctors use it to determine the severity of scoliosis and to devise appropriate treatment plans for patients.

Doctors look at the spine on a front-to-back X-ray, then they measure the curvature based on the end or "transitional" vertebrae. These specific vertebrae are the top and bottom vertebrae that are affected by the spine's abnormal curvature. To determine the Cobb angle measurement, a line is drawn from the top of the *superior* vertebrae, and another is drawn from the bottom end of the *inferior* vertebrae. Eventually, these two lines meet and form an angle, which is known as the Cobb angle.

C-shaped curves are relatively straightforward to measure in this manner. However, when it comes to S-shaped curvatures (those that are made up of two curves), doctors will adapt by using the bottom vertebrae of the upper curve as the top vertebrae of the lower curve.

The Cobb angle measurement is the standard doctors use to evaluate and measure scoliosis, but it is far from perfect. For one thing, it imposes a two-dimensional viewpoint on what is a three-dimensional condition. In other words, this measurement only provides a fraction of the full picture. It doesn't tell the whole story in terms of what is going on with a patient's spine.

To truly measure and analyze the abnormal curvature of a spine properly, it's necessary to combine X-rays with other types of evaluations and scans. The twists and turns that may be present in a scoliotic spine won't appear in a basic X-ray. Yes, the X-ray is a fantastic tool that can tell us a lot about what's going on with a patient's spine. But in order to treat scoliosis effectively, it is necessary to understand the spine's curvature from a number of different angles and perspectives.

To me, the Cobb angle is a starting point. If the angle measures more than ten degrees, it means that scoliosis, by definition, is present. But that's not nearly enough information to go by when it comes to designing an effective treatment plan to reduce the spine's curvature. I use the Cobb angle measurement as just one factor—an important factor, to be sure, but just one of many.

Another imperfection of the Cobb angle measurement is that it's often inconsistent. It doesn't offer a precise measurement; in fact, there is a significant margin of error involved. That's why if you see ten different doctors, you'll probably receive ten different Cobb angle measurements. What's more, patients aren't always placed the same for their X-rays. So two different X-rays taken at two different times could reveal differences. Altogether, the variables involved in measuring a Cobb angle can account for as much as a five-degree difference from doctor to doctor.

A five-degree difference might not seem like much, but consider the ten-degree designation for scoliosis. One doctor may measure a curvature at eight degrees, while another measures it at thirteen degrees. It's the same person with the same spine, but one measurement is an indicator of scoliosis, while the other is not. With early detection and proactive treatment being so important, patients cannot rely on these inconsistent measurements alone to determine how they should move forward.

Why Does Adult Scoliosis Develop in the First Place?

It is quite natural for you to be curious about the origins of your condition if you've been diagnosed with scoliosis. Sadly, most scoliosis patients will never know the exact conditions that led to the development of their abnormal spinal curvatures. On a personal level, scoliosis in adults can be incredibly frustrating because it presents so many unanswerable questions.

The fact is that if you've been diagnosed with idiopathic scoliosis, no amount of investigation or medical sleuthing will reveal the reasons why you developed the condition. The term *idiopathic* means that there is literally no known or discoverable cause. It's a tough fact to acknowledge for many adults. Patients are routinely flabbergasted when they decide to look for answers, only to be told that it's unlikely that they will ever find them.

In children, idiopathic scoliosis is usually detected at age ten or older—if it's detected at all. These cases affect about four percent of children, with girls typically showing more pronounced abnormal curvatures than boys. In the earliest stages of the condition when curvatures are small, scoliosis affects boys and girls about equally. But over time, the ratio of girls to boys increases.

We also know that the percentage of adults with ASA is higher than four percent, which means that significant numbers of people with scoliosis aren't being diagnosed in adolescence. This is either because they aren't being examined for the condition, or it's because the curvature when tested is so subtle as to be undetectable. Again, scoliosis is a progressive condition; there's no getting around that fact. For this reason, subtle cases only become more serious over time. So if you showed no signs of scoliosis as a teenager, but now have a detectable abnormal curvature, it's possible that you've been living with scoliosis for longer than you think.

It may surprise you to know that so much about scoliosis is unknown. This can be frustrating, I know. In our culture, we tend to demand answers for our problems, and it's reasonable to expect to find them, given the technology and resources we all have at our disposal. But when it comes to scoliosis, patients often must treat their condition without ever knowing what may have caused it.

Even for adults who have the De Novo—or the degenerative—form of the condition, answers aren't so clear cut. Yes, we know that degeneration of the spine through aging is the dominant underlying cause. However, the precise mechanics of its development is still somewhat mysterious.

You probably have some questions at this point:

- *Does it really matter what type of adult scoliosis I have?*
- *Could I have prevented my scoliosis from developing or progressing?*
- *If early detection is so important for treating scoliosis, is it too late for me?*

So, does it matter what type of adult scoliosis you have? Yes and no. Regardless of the type of scoliosis an adult patient has, the treatment must go beyond the symptoms to address the underlying causes of those symptoms.

On one hand, understanding the type of adult scoliosis a patient has can provide insight and clarity; people feel better, especially in our culture, when they can arrive at answers to their problems, as I mentioned previously. On the other hand, the appropriate treatment plan for an individual patient will always need to be developed for that specific person, regardless of the cause of scoliosis or how it developed over time. Each body—and each spine—is completely unique, so effective treatment needs to take this into consideration.

If you're wondering whether you could have prevented your adult scoliosis from developing or progressing, I can understand why you may be scanning your past to look for answers. It's natural and completely human to do so. The truth is that, yes, if you and your family had had the knowledge and awareness of your condition at that time, perhaps the condition could have been treated sooner. But it's also possible that if you had been diagnosed in adolescence, you would have been put on the traditional treatment path of watching and waiting until your curve got so severe that it required surgery. Now that you're an adult with awareness of your condition, you can make different choices for yourself than may have been made for you when you were younger. You don't have to watch and wait, nor do you have to prepare yourself for the inevitability of surgery. You can seek treatment to reduce the abnormal curvature of your spine without surgery.

If you're concerned about early detection, consider this: What if you had waited even longer to seek relief from your pain and discomfort? We cannot go back in time to diagnose cases of scoliosis with the knowledge we have now; we can only work with what we know right now. An adult diagnosis of scoliosis can make it seem like you missed the boat on early detection, but that's no reason to despair. The important point to keep in mind is that you have already begun to take proactive steps to make your life and health better. While it would have been nice to be able to treat your scoliosis earlier in life, all you can do is what's best right now.

A diagnosis of scoliosis as an adult can seem hopeless, but I'm here to tell you that there's ample reason to remain hopeful. We know more about adult scoliosis today than we ever have in the condition's history. New approaches to treatment that don't involve surgery are becoming increasingly available. Every day, more and more scoliosis success stories are written by people just like you. They thought they were resigned to an adulthood marked by pain and exhaustion. But the diagnosis of scoliosis gave them validation and a reason to move forward with hope.

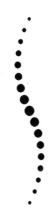

CHAPTER THREE

How Is Adult Scoliosis Different from Adolescent Idiopathic Scoliosis?

AS YOU ENDEAVOR TO understand more about the condition of your spine and how it impacts your life, you might be frustrated to learn that adults like you aren't discussed as often or in as much detail as your youthful counterparts.

I have to admit that when my colleagues and I discuss scoliosis, we tend to focus on adolescents who have the condition. And if you look at any literature related to scoliosis—or if you perform a simple Google search on the condition—you will notice that adults are rarely mentioned. If people above the age of eighteen are discussed with regard to scoliosis, they are typically presented as an afterthought.

But consider this: Without treatment or intervention, every adolescent with scoliosis eventually becomes an adult with scoliosis. So even though teenagers may be the focus of most scoliosis discussions and literature, adults are also impacted considerably by the condition. In fact, I would argue that adults with scoliosis experience greater challenges than teens.

Both adults and adolescents with scoliosis experience challenges associated with their appearance and other aesthetic concerns. Honestly, teens probably feel this impact more sensitively than adults, given the pressures they feel to fit in and find a comfortable place, socially. Teens just want to feel "normal," but scoliosis makes them unique in ways that aren't always positive for their social lives. Typically, adults don't feel the intense social pressures that teens experience. But that doesn't mean people your age stop caring about how their clothes fit or how they appear to others. Being stylish and having an aesthetically pleasing appearance is important in adulthood, and scoliosis can get in the way of a person's ideal image of themselves.

Adults and adolescents with the condition also must deal with the fact that scoliosis is progressive in nature. For teenagers who have developing bodies and minds, the progression of their scoliosis (and the potential associated health concerns) is usually not a huge concern. If you have (or have had) teenage children, you know that the worldview of an adolescent is a lot different from that of an adult. They feel invincible, or that nothing can stop them from achieving their dreams. Nevertheless, teenagers are highly emotional creatures who are usually far more thoughtful about these things than adults give them credit for.

For adults, progression of scoliosis makes treating the condition continuously more urgent. As the scoliosis becomes more severe, it puts greater pressure on the body's organs and systems, often leading to health issues that, on the surface, would seem to have nothing to do with the spine. If you're an adult with scoliosis, I'm sure you've received all sorts of advice regarding your symptoms, none of which has addressed the real underlying issue. This is, unfortunately, pretty normal for people in your position.

Adults and adolescents who have scoliosis must both deal with the progressive nature of the condition. And they both have concerns about appearances and aesthetics. This is where the similarities end. Adolescents with scoliosis may believe that their experience will remain more or less the same throughout life, but there are significant differences between scoliosis as a teen and having the condition in adulthood.

The most notable difference is a four-letter word we all dread: *pain.*

When I see adult patients who have been living with scoliosis since adolescence, they often ask me how the condition can be so painful in adulthood when it caused virtually no pain in their younger years. It doesn't make sense to them. This is when I remind them that scoliosis is a progressive condition. If they have done nothing to treat it since adolescence, it has not been sitting idle in the body; it was progressing all along. And the greater the abnormal curvature, the greater the likelihood that it will cause pain somewhere in the body.

Interestingly, it isn't uncommon for me to treat children with eighty-degree curvatures who experience no pain. But I'll treat a forty-year-old patient who has a thirty-degree curve that causes severe pain. Why is this the case? All eighty degrees of the child's curvature happened during the time of growth and development, which prevents the compression of the spine. And it is the compression of the spine that tends to cause pain. For the adult, they may have experienced a minor curvature in adolescence, but in adulthood, that curve grew slowly but significantly relative to their curve at a time when the growth cycle had already stopped. Therefore, compression of the spine is present in the adult, which is why the condition causes so much more pain.

Scoliosis is also kinder to growing bodies, with regard to pain. As I mentioned previously, the growth of the human body in adolescence stretches the spine upward, relieving the compression and associated pain that would otherwise occur. This is the main reason why pain is so rare in adolescent scoliosis patients. It's also a major reason why it feels okay to simply watch and wait instead of proactively treating the condition.

It's very common for me to encounter adult patients who resent that they were told to watch and wait when they were younger. They had no idea how much physical pain the condition would eventually cause. In fact, they were just following the guidance of the medical professionals and experts they went to see at the time. But then their bodies stopped growing and the aches and pains began to accumulate—slowly, at first, and barely noticeable. By middle age, though, adults who have scoliosis typically experience symptoms that affect their back, hips, legs, or other areas of the body. It's painful—extremely so in some cases—and it has a tendency to use up every ounce of energy a person has.

The pain of scoliosis is bad enough. But that's not the only thing adults with the condition have to deal with. While adolescents can feel free and experience life without many limitations, adults become exhausted by the condition quite quickly. Pain leads to exhaustion, which leads to a loss of freedom. If you are an adult with scoliosis, I bet that you have had to limit your life in ways that don't feel comfortable. You've had to eliminate activities that you love, and you may have become increasingly dependent upon others.

Because scoliosis is a progressive condition, this scenario only becomes more troubling as time goes on. For many adults with scoliosis, the condition has become so severe that they lose their ability to walk or even stand. Decades of gravity's impact have caused postural collapse, and for these patients, it becomes necessary to depend on others because of their disability.

If you're holding out hope that your scoliosis may pause or stabilize on its own, I have to warn you that this never happens. Scoliosis never improves by itself or without intervention. It may move slowly, but it is always moving, just like the turtle in its race against the hare.

It's a situation that can make you feel powerless, especially if the only advice you have heard from experts is to watch and wait.

The fact is that the progression of a scoliosis curve in an adult's spine will be as much as three degrees a year, depending on a number of factors. This is true even if you entered adulthood with a minor abnormal curvature. The rate at which your scoliosis progresses cannot be determined, but know this: it will definitely progress. It's not because you're unlucky or that you did anything wrong. It's simply the nature of the condition. That's why I always recommend taking action instead of watching and waiting.

Why is scoliosis so unrelentingly progressive? What is it that makes it always get worse over time? One word—*gravity*. Gravity may not seem like the strongest force, but it's consistent and patient. There isn't a day that goes by when your spine is unaffected by gravity. Over time, the effects of gravity take their toll. And as long as gravity continues to exist, it will always have an unkind impact on anything that bears the load of the body—like the spine of someone who has scoliosis.

Adult scoliosis shares much in common with adolescent scoliosis, but the way it impacts a person's life is much different. For adults like you, relief from pain, stiffness, and exhaustion becomes a higher priority with each passing day. You should think about next steps in a serious way right now, with the intention of taking action.

So what should you do next? I'll explore your options in the next chapter.

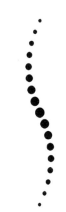

CHAPTER FOUR

Where Will Your Scoliosis Journey Take You Next?

ALMOST EVERY ADULT WITH scoliosis reaches the point where you are right now: fed up with the ever-increasing pain of your condition and scared about their ability to live a full, healthy and active life. Can anything be done? Will you have to have an expensive, invasive spinal surgery? Will your condition reduce not only your quality of life, but your life expectancy?

What we know for sure is that doing nothing doesn't work. Taking no action will only allow your spine to move further and further away from a normal, healthy curvature. Your pain will increase while your mobility decreases. When I talk about the progression of scoliosis, this is what I mean. At this point in your life—and your journey with scoliosis—the turtle has caught up to the hare; you can no longer assume that you have plenty of time to act before the condition becomes too severe.

Sadly, the traditional set of options for adults with scoliosis leaves a lot to be desired.

Basically, the established medical model for treating scoliosis will tell you that these are your options:

1. Do nothing (i.e., watch and wait)
2. Focus on the conditions or symptoms that arise from scoliosis without treating the scoliosis
3. Undergo surgery

If you take a closer look at these options, you'll notice that they either dance around the issue (options one and two) or they take, in my opinion, an extreme course of action (option three). You will also notice that they all work together. Doing nothing leaves you in a situation where the symptoms become increasingly severe, so you treat those just to find some amount of relief. Meanwhile, your spine will continue to grow away from its normal curvature. Eventually, your abnormal spinal curvature will progress to a severe curve, more than fifty degrees, and doctors will probably tell you that you've become a candidate for surgery.

The do-nothing, watch-and-wait approach is the standard today, as it has been for decades. It is an established model that people are reluctant to question since it has been the top treatment option for so long. But does it work? Yes, it works amazingly well for putting people on the path to surgery. It doesn't work well in terms of its ability to prevent the continuing progression of your spine's abnormal curvature. In fact, it fails in that regard.

I have talked to and treated many adults who were told, as children, that they wouldn't have to worry about scoliosis in adulthood. Some of them were even told that it wouldn't worsen. There is absolutely no evidence to suggest that this is true. In fact, the opposite is true. These badly mistaken beliefs persist because the watch-and-wait approach has become so deeply ingrained into the traditional treatment approach.

Watching and waiting may have seemed like a reasonable approach for dealing with your scoliosis if you were diagnosed when you were younger. The condition didn't affect you nearly as much as it does now. You weren't in pain like you are now, either. So now that you're an adult, it becomes critical that you ignore the advice to watch and wait. You can receive treatment right now that helps you prevent the continuing progression of your scoliosis and relieves your pain. The longer you wait, though, the more difficult it will be to reduce your curvature and ease your discomfort.

As you watch and wait, your symptoms will become more severe. Your pain level will rise, and your energy level will drop. These changes may happen slowly over the course of many years, but they are inevitable. And these are just the physical realities of watching and waiting with scoliosis. Your emotional and mental health is likely to become weakened as you wait to take action. Because you're likely to experience an increase in pain and discomfort as your condition progresses, you'll probably feel uncomfortable emotions like fear and anxiety begin to become more prominent in your life. And when your mental health takes a downturn, it often manifests by creating even more physical symptoms to deal with. It's a vicious cycle.

Seeking relief in this scenario usually means treating the symptoms of your condition without addressing their underlying causes. So adults will seek relief by going to yoga classes or visiting massage therapists. I have nothing against yoga or massage in a general sense. Anything that helps the average person—with the average body—relieve stress and improve function is a good thing. However, when these treatments are presented as legitimate options for relieving the pain and progression of scoliosis, I have to push back strongly.

Certainly, yoga and massage can provide temporary relief from the symptoms of adult scoliosis. But I see too many patients allowing their curvatures to progress as they continue to get nothing more than short-term, Band-Aid solutions. In the best-case scenario, yoga and massage will provide a little bit of relief for a few days. In the worst-case scenario, these modalities will provide no relief while putting extra stress and strain on the body. This leads to even greater levels of pain. Again, yoga and massage do nothing to reduce abnormal spinal curvatures from scoliosis. You may think that all you have to do is practice yoga consistently, and the temporary relief you feel may be extended. The reality is that your temporary relief doesn't indicate that your scoliosis has been resolved in any way. You may not be able to feel the pain from scoliosis immediately after a massage or yoga session, but the condition is still there, and the pain will always return.

Many adults with scoliosis also wonder about traditional gym exercises. Is it possible to strengthen the body and relieve the pain of scoliosis by lifting weights, rowing, biking, or doing high-intensity interval training? The thing to understand about these types of exercises is that they are dynamic muscle movers. They are great for building up your biceps and other larger muscle groups, which are known as type-two muscles. The muscles we want to address when working with adults with scoliosis are type one. They function more with regard to the body's endurance. Consider your ability to hold good posture. The muscle fibers involved are type one, which require long, slow, constant contraction, which is absolutely *not* what you're getting when you go to the gym.

Yoga, massage, and gym exercise are all examples of things adults with scoliosis do to treat their symptoms. Doing this might feel good, but as you treat your symptoms, your scoliosis will only continue to progress steadily. As it progresses, it's likely to cause increasing amounts of pain, no matter what kind of exercise, yoga, or massage routine you may be involved in.

If exercise or milder, more "natural" methods of treating scoliosis symptoms fail to deliver results, many adults with the condition will turn to pain pills. First, they try over-the-counter remedies. But then those medications begin to lose their effectiveness as the condition progresses and causes increasing amounts of pain. At this point, patients often ask their doctors for ever-stronger prescriptions. This can lead to dependence and addiction. Doctors are simply doing their jobs when they prescribe medications—they are trained extensively in medicine, which is why they prescribe medicine as the solution for so many issues. Unfortunately, this is a path that is all too familiar for adults who struggle with physical pain in our culture. For those who have scoliosis, the pain tends to persist or grow worse, all while the spine's abnormal curvature continues its progression. How much medication will you need to move your spine into its normal position with its normal curvature? Sadly, no amount of medication can improve scoliosis. This is just another example of treating the symptoms versus treating the underlying conditions that cause them.

Because pain—and pain management—is such a major factor for adults with scoliosis, I'll go into much more detail on the subject in the next section of this book. But for now, it's important to know that you can do so much more than simply manage your pain. It's possible to address and relieve your pain by getting to the structural root of your condition. After years of living with ever-increasing pain, I know that it seems like you need to keep lowering your expectations of what is possible. But there are non-invasive, nonsurgical treatments available today that relieve the intense pain of scoliosis by actually reducing the abnormal spinal curvature.

For now, though, let's continue looking at the path you're likely to take if you treat your scoliosis using the orthopedic, surgical model.

Under the traditional scoliosis treatment model, surgery is presented as the final gate patients must pass through in order to receive the relief they are so desperate for. It is also a last resort. When patients reach this point, they're in so much pain and discomfort that risky, invasive, and expensive surgery can seem like a godsend. They have been living lives marked by hopelessness; surgery offers a glimmer of hope.

Spinal surgeons are amazing at their jobs. They are well trained, highly skilled, and very knowledgeable. They perform numerous surgeries every year, and most of them have an extremely high "success" rate. They can make something as serious as surgery seem like it's no big deal. But surgery should only ever be a person's last resort.

Surgery is expensive. If you are a person with an average income, it represents the kind of expense that can change your life—and not in a good way. If surgery worked well, I can see why the cost would be worth it. But surgery doesn't always work well. It may stabilize the spine, but it isn't likely to reduce an abnormal scoliosis curvature. Certainly, surgeons will always attempt to reduce the scoliosis, but that doesn't necessarily lead to greater health or spine function. Ultimately, patients must ask themselves if it's all worth the cost—not just in financial terms, but at the cost of losing mobility or function. And in the vast majority of cases, fusion leads to the loss of spinal function. A straight spine that is fused doesn't equal greater function, so attempts to straighten it should always serve the larger purpose of improving function.

When a person with scoliosis has spinal-fusion surgery, it also removes a number of far less invasive options off of the table. In my practice, for example, I can work with virtually anyone, regardless of age or curvature, to reduce the impact of their scoliosis. But once they have had surgery, many of the techniques and procedures I utilize become more difficult and less predictable. Surgery may seem promising, but I believe that it only brings patients closer to a point of no return.

To many patients, scoliosis surgery represents the end of the road. They see it as the end of their suffering and the conclusion of a story that has haunted them for most of their adult lives. They envision and idealize their lives after surgery, believing that they are about to get a new lease on life. Sometimes, patients do find that their lives are better after surgery. But the risk of a failed scoliosis surgery increases with age, and there's no guarantee that surgery will provide relief, even when it's done perfectly.

To me, when a patient has spinal-fusion surgery for scoliosis, it doesn't mean the end of the road. Rather, it means that the patient has turned down an entirely new road, with its own set of twists, turns, and bumps. Patients can be so enamored of their idealized life postsurgery, that they fail to consider the possible complications of going under the knife. The fact is that surgery doesn't always relieve a patient's pain. The spine can also fail to fuse, causing a condition known as *pseudoarthosis*. Surgery also opens up the possibility of infection or major blood loss. Complications can also arise many months or even years down the road. I can understand why an adult who has been living in pain for decades would seek relief via surgery. I just want to make sure people know that it isn't necessarily the solution they think it is. There are other, less risky, less expensive, and less invasive options.

The three traditional scoliosis treatment options I have outlined in this chapter aren't very appealing, are they? Turns out they aren't very effective either. So why are these considered the best available options under the traditional scoliosis treatment model?

I cannot speak for the medical establishment and its standards of treatment for scoliosis. The status quo for traditional treatment has been well established, and it's rarely been questioned, so it makes sense that it remains the dominant model for treatment.

What I *can* speak for is what I know through decades of experience, education, practice, and getting to know countless people with scoliosis: hope is possible. You don't have to endure more years of misery just so you can be deemed a candidate for spinal surgery.

It breaks my heart to see what adult scoliosis patients go through. Year after year, they feel the increasing effects of their condition and its almost exponential impact on their bodies. They live in so much pain and discomfort that surgery seems appealing. Anything to give the possibility of some relief.

It's heartbreaking to me because I know what is possible when adults with scoliosis receive treatment that addresses the condition at its core. I have seen adult patients relieve their pain and regain active, healthy lives—all without surgery. You don't have to watch and wait. You don't have to prepare yourself for the inevitably of surgery. You can take action now.

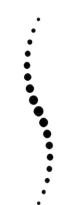

The Pain of Adult Scoliosis

PAIN IS A MAJOR characteristic of adult scoliosis—and the most likely factor to influence an adult to become proactive about the condition.

In children and adolescents, the absence of severe pain is actually used as an indicator to help doctors determine that the patient has idiopathic scoliosis. If strong levels of pain are present in these younger patients, it usually indicates that an underlying health issue is the culprit. But typically, scoliosis will only cause mild-to-moderate pain in adolescent patients, if it causes pain at all.

For adults, strong, challenging pain goes hand in hand with scoliosis more often than not.

Naturally, when people think about the type of pain that might be caused by scoliosis, they consider how it affects the body. Physical pain from scoliosis in an adult can be excruciating. It's often the factor that spurs patients into action after years of inaction.

Physical pain isn't the only consideration, however.

Scoliosis in adulthood can lead to emotional pain as well. We are accustomed to considering the emotions of adolescents who have scoliosis, because they live in emotional pressure cookers anyway. School, relationships, status, planning for the future, and managing scoliosis is a lot. So parents and doctors usually do a good job of helping teens cope.

Adults don't share the same stresses and strains as adolescents, but that doesn't mean they are emotionless creatures. As you know, emotions in adulthood may not be as intense on the surface level as they are in adolescence. But they are much deeper and more complex. Therefore, scoliosis can have a major emotional impact on adults too, adding to the already troubling aspects of physical pain.

In this section, I will describe the realities of physical and emotional pain for adults with scoliosis. I will also describe the ways in which adult patients can find actual relief from the pain caused by scoliosis. Finally, I will go into greater detail about what your life can look like as you work to address the structural issues that form the foundation of your pain.

CHAPTER FIVE

Physical Pain from Scoliosis

IT WOULDN'T SURPRISE ME to know that you're reading this book because you are in pain.

As I have mentioned previously in this book, pain is the great motivator for adults who have scoliosis. Adults in our society can put up with quite a bit in their lives. The average American, for example, lives a highly stressed life.

According to Gallup (https://news.gallup.com/poll/249098/ americans-stress-worry-anger-intensified-2018.aspx), 55 percent of Americans experience stress during an average day. If that doesn't seem high, consider that the world average is just 35 percent. In fact, the only country more stressed out than the United States is Greece, where 59 percent of the population reported feeling stressed. If we look a little closer at the numbers, the age group that's affected most by stress is the thirty-to-forty-nine category. This age range also happens to be the time frame when adults with scoliosis tend to reach a tipping point in terms of their ability to cope with the condition and its associated pain. Sixty-five percent of people in this particular age group experience stress on a regular basis. People over fifty tend to be less stressed, but still, nearly half of that group (44 percent) feels stress regularly as well.

As if that weren't enough, women tend to be more stressed out than men. According to a study by the American Psychological Association (https://www.apa.org/news/press/releases/stress/2014/stress-report.pdf), the average woman reports a stress level of 5.1 on a scale of one to ten. Men report an average stress level of 4.4.

Statistically, this is important information when it comes to understanding the impact adult scoliosis can have on an individual.

Individuals in our society experience more stress on a daily basis than people almost anywhere else in the world. Furthermore, the most stressed-out people in our country are those who fall squarely in the age range where adult scoliosis would begin to cause undeniable pain. And women—who are more likely to have adult scoliosis than men—also experience significantly more stress than their male counterparts.

Stress would be considered an aspect of emotional pain, and I will certainly discuss it in more detail in the next chapter. But I believe you cannot have a discussion about physical pain without addressing the conditions under which it thrives. Stress creates conditions in the body that make it easy for physical pain to manifest and spread. And usually, people don't seek relief until they reach the point where physical pain begins to limit their lives. They will put up with unprecedented levels of stress, but they cannot deal with the pain. That says something about the level of pain patients must be in by the time they start looking for relief and answers.

Adults with scoliosis can experience physical pain in numerous areas of the body. Pain can exist in places that might seem to have nothing to do with the spine. That is why patients receive misdiagnoses so often. Sometimes, patients experience symptoms like headaches or tingling in the extremities. Scoliosis is a condition of the spine that can potentially affect the entire body, so it's important to follow symptoms to their structural root. Otherwise, you're just delaying the inevitable: Eventually, you will need to address your scoliosis one way or another.

In this chapter, I will describe the most common types of pain that adult scoliosis patients experience.

Whether you have adolescent idiopathic scoliosis in an adult (ASA) or De Novo scoliosis, you are highly likely to experience significant physical pain.

Pain that comes from physical activity is more common among those with scoliosis than it is among those without. This is why you may tend to feel worn out or exhausted after minimal time spent engaging in activities. The reason for this is that the spine's degeneration is accompanied by a reduction in water content in the spinal disks. This creates conditions that lead to greater inflammation. Pinched nerves might arise from this set of circumstances, too, along with disk bulges and herniations. Additionally, patients can experience pain from the development of arthritis in the facet joints.

Spinal stenosis is a common condition among adults with scoliosis, particularly those who have the degenerative, De Novo form. This condition, which is a narrowing of the spinal canal, creates a wide range of issues in the body, many of which lead to increased pain. The condition is brought on by inflammation such as the thickening of ligaments or disk bulges. Nerves are made to pass through narrower and narrower passages, which leads to compression, which, in turn, leads to cramping, tingling, and increased pain.

Being upright can place more pressure on the spine and make the spinal canal even narrower. That's why sitting and resting, or even bending forward temporarily, can relieve the pain associated with spinal stenosis. These actions actually contribute to a natural expansion of the spinal canal, which is why they can feel so relieving for back pain.

Back pain, whether it's caused by spinal stenosis or not, is quite common in adults who have scoliosis. It makes perfect sense that the condition would lead to pain in the spine, since it's a condition of the spine. If you have experienced an increase in back pain, it could be because of adult scoliosis and its progression.

Scoliosis in adults doesn't just cause pain in the back, though.

Often, adults with scoliosis will experience more significant pain in one of their shoulders than they feel in their backs. This is typical.

Perhaps you've felt minor back pain but have been experiencing more significant pain in one shoulder. Likely, it's the shoulder on the side of your body where your ribs are more prominent. When your spine curves to the right, it can cause shoulder pain on the right side of the body. This happens because the body is trying to compensate and move your spine back into its normal position; tendons and muscles stretch and work overtime, creating stress, tension, and pain.

Shoulder pain usually progresses at the same rate of the scoliosis progression. It will begin in one shoulder, but it almost always moves to the opposite shoulder if the scoliosis isn't addressed. The opposite shoulder—the one away from the direction of your curvature—experiences an imbalance that increases as the torso twists, leading to increasing amounts of pain and discomfort.

Pain in one or more shoulders from scoliosis should not be ignored. It will never go away on its own. Nor is there anything you can do to your shoulders, specifically, that will make the pain subside. The shoulder pain you experience is a side effect of your ever-progressing scoliosis, so it's necessary to treat the underlying condition in order to have a positive impact on your pain.

Hip pain is also fairly common among adults with scoliosis.

You may or may not experience pain in the hips from scoliosis. Though it's common, it is less common than back or shoulder pain in adults with the condition. Nevertheless, you should be aware that pain in this region is likely an indicator of the progression of your scoliosis.

Scoliosis can lead to an unbalanced posture. Sometimes, this manifests with the pelvic bones on one side of the body appearing higher than the other while standing. If this is the case, it's only a matter of time before the imbalance leads to physical pain in the hips.

Standing or walking for extended periods of time will bring out this type of pain. Gravity is a major culprit here, which is why it can feel so relieving to sit or lie down. Unbalanced posture also puts more strain on the body, which can lead to further degeneration of the hip joints.

If your hips are tilted from your scoliosis, the lack of balance means one hip takes on a larger workload than its counterpart on the other side of the body. This can cause a chain reaction of conditions that arise from asymmetrical overuse of the muscles and tendons. Rest may make you feel like this pain has gone away. Unfortunately, it always returns. It only gets worse over time.

As I mentioned previously in this book, scoliosis in adults can also be the cause of painful headaches. That is because the condition can cause a muscle imbalance in the shoulders and neck, which can lead to headaches. In fact, almost half of all headaches come from problems in the neck.

The neck-and-shoulder region of your body contains a complex web of muscles that connect to the muscles in the base of your head. Tension and inflammation from scoliosis can cause pains in these areas. The postural strain caused by scoliosis can lead to increased tension in these muscle groups, putting pressure on the nerves and creating conditions under which tension headaches thrive. Of course, the usual stresses and strains of adult life can also contribute to headaches. Stress, depression, and anxiety are all contributors to tension in the neck, head, and shoulders, so if you experience any of these issues, you're more likely to suffer from painful headaches. Furthermore, if your job requires you to sit and stare at a screen for several hours each day, it only increases the odds that you'll experience headaches.

Scoliosis, Stenosis, and Sciatica

I have already briefly explained the relationship between scoliosis and stenosis, but I feel like it deserves some special attention. Basically, it describes the narrowing of the spinal canal due to events like degeneration, inflammation, and the development of bone spurs. Stenosis can also occur due to misalignment: scoliosis is always related to rotation, and the rotation can create a misalignment that places a vertebra out of position, thus causing a stenosis between the two spinal bones (*see graphic*). When the large openings of the thirty-three vertebrae become narrow, it puts pressure on the spinal cord, which can lead to a host of issues and a great deal of physical pain.

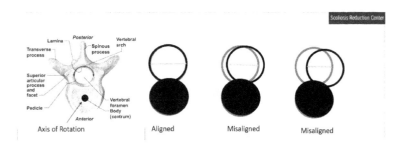

There are actually more openings in the spine known as *spinal foramen*. These openings allow nerves to extend from the spinal cord out to other parts of the body like the arms and legs. When these smaller openings become narrow, the condition is known as *foraminal stenosis*.

Foramen size can be reduced drastically through a range of factors. Arthritis can lead to the production of bone spurs that exist within these narrow openings, causing them to become even narrower, which puts pressure on the nerves that travel there. Subluxation, which is another word for the misalignment of the spine, also reduces the size of foramen.

Your spinal cord is an incredibly important part of your body. So forcing it to exist in an increasingly narrow space creates impacts that can be felt all over your body. Physical pain, numbness, and weakness can become evident. Burning and tingling sensations may be felt as well, alongside the uncomfortable feeling of pins and needles in the arms and legs. In some cases, spinal stenosis can even lead to a loss of motor control.

Sciatica, which usually only affects one side of a patient's lower body, is another painful condition that commonly affects adults with scoliosis.

The term *sciatica* is derived from the sciatic nerve, which runs from the lower back down the length of each leg. It can be caused by stenosis or other factors that irritate or compress the nerve roots in the lower spine region. It comes with many unfortunate symptoms too, including the aforementioned pain, numbness, tingling, and burning. Certain pains that accompany sciatica worsen when sitting. Other types of pain from sciatica can make it difficult to stand up.

As you can surely imagine, sciatica is a serious issue for adults who have scoliosis. It can become a constant, painful companion, especially for adults with scoliosis who are also overweight, have unsupportive mattresses to sleep on, or live sedentary lifestyles.

Another factor that can contribute to your sciatic symptoms: wearing high heels.

Whether it's through stenosis, sciatica, some other symptom, or a combination of them, adult scoliosis will always lead to painful complications that seem to stack on top of each other. This is just more reason for you to be proactive about treating your scoliosis.

Pelvic pain often accompanies scoliosis, too. Have you heard of something in your body called the sacroiliac joint? Not many people have, but it's a crucial area of the body to understand if you want to get to the bottom of your scoliosis pain.

If you look at the pelvic girdle, which is a fairly complex system, you will notice that the sacrum, or tailbone, connects to pelvic bones on the right and left sides. These connections form the sacroiliac joints. When there is either too much or too little movement of these joints, inflammation can occur, leading to potentially debilitating pain. Scoliosis can cause this type of imbalance because it tends to force the patient to tilt the body to one side, putting extra weight and pressure on the pelvic joints.

When the sacroiliac joints are affected by scoliosis, it can lead to pain in the pelvis, of course, but inflammation of these joints can lead to lower back pain or sacral pain as well. In addition, you may experience pain that runs down the back of your legs (also known as *sciatica*) and other issues such as an increase in urinary frequency, difficult walking, sitting, or standing, or even numbness in your extremities.

Since the lumbo-pelvic region of the body serves as a hub for your nervous system, numerous connections are made here. That makes it especially vulnerable to the effects of scoliosis. Because of the interconnection of nerves in this area, inflammation can cause pain and discomfort in several different regions of the body.

It really depends on each individual patient how sacroiliac joints will affect the manner in which scoliosis impacts the body.

Adults with scoliosis feel the condition much differently than adolescents. Adolescents must endure a number of challenges, but physical pain is usually not one of them. For adults, pain is, by far, the number one factor that motivates them to seek treatment. It can be intense and excruciating, so much so that it causes adults with scoliosis to miss out on the good things in life.

Thankfully, adults with scoliosis don't have to simply endure their ever-increasing physical pain. They don't have to rely on pain pills or other Band-Aid treatments, either. The best way to treat physical pain for those who have adult scoliosis is to address their structural issues directly.

There is reason to have hope when it comes to experiencing relief from your physical pain.

But what about the emotional pain that tends to come with adult scoliosis? The next chapter dives right into this important, but often overlooked, side of the pain equation.

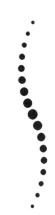

CHAPTER SIX

The Emotional Pain of Scoliosis

IN THE PREVIOUS CHAPTER, I spent some time describing how scoliosis can contribute to headaches and other pains in the neck, head, and shoulder regions. Headaches can also manifest from experiencing emotional issues such as stress, anxiety or depression.

In reality, scoliosis is almost as much an emotional condition as it is a physical one. And its emotional impacts can contribute to the physical challenges—and vice versa.

While scoliosis is a structural condition of the spine, recognizing its emotional impact is crucial for aiding treatment and recovery. Focusing solely on the body ignores the deep emotional layers of the condition, which must also be addressed in order to treat scoliosis successfully.

There's a lot of talk about the emotional impact of scoliosis on teenagers, for good reason. As you know, adolescents are highly emotional creatures, even when they're perfectly healthy in a physical sense. When scoliosis is added to the mix, already complex emotional states become even more heightened and complicated.

The emotional roller coaster that teens find themselves on under normal circumstances just gets scarier when an adolescent has to deal with scoliosis on top of it all.

Sadly, when patients turn eighteen and become adults, there's a tendency to stop paying attention to the emotional impacts of the condition. We focus so much on physical pain because it is, by far, the primary reason adults with the condition usually come to see doctors or chiropractors like me for treatment. And we also tend to assume that adults always have their emotions under control and require no help in dealing with them in a healthy manner.

You and I both know that this just isn't the case.

It's important for you to understand that strong emotions are often found accompanying cases of adult scoliosis. The impact on your emotional life will be profound, often surprisingly so. But this is quite normal, and it's nothing to be afraid of. You must rise to the challenge of understanding and confronting those emotions, though, if you want to work through them successfully as part of your treatment.

Scoliosis, being a progressive condition, only gets worse over time. Therefore, if you have been watching and waiting for a while, you've probably received worse and worse news each time you have gone in to be examined. You may be used to this reality by now, but you should also give yourself the grace to recognize that receiving so much negative news has had an emotional impact. The fact is that scoliosis patients—adults especially—aren't used to receiving good news with regard to their condition. This can wear a person down, even without them knowing it.

Chances are that you've received very little good news about your scoliosis since your diagnosis. Or if you've not been diagnosed, but suspect that you have the condition, you've probably not been taken seriously. This also has an extremely negative impact on one's emotional state.

When you have a serious medical condition that causes increasing amounts of pain and exhaustion, staying upbeat, positive, and present can seem impossible. Add to this scenario the fact that you can't seem to find relief, and it creates a pressure cooker of stress, pain, and exhaustion that can lead to severe emotional difficulty.

From what I've observed, the treatment path a patient takes can have a great impact on emotions. Under the traditional, orthopedic model, surgery is the end goal and last resort. Adult patients who seek relief under this model of treatment often feel a mixed set of emotions. On one hand, they feel like they can look forward to a surgical solution to their problems. Surgery, they are told, will provide relief and serve as an endpoint to a painful journey.

On the other hand, adult patients understand that surgery is inherently risky. It's also incredibly invasive and expensive. On an emotional level, the prospect of surgery, while somewhat promising in some ways, can cause a great deal of anxiety and stress. Additionally, there's ample research showing that scoliosis surgery can create negative psychological effects. This study, for example, reveals that those who have undergone spinal-fusion surgery involving Harrington rods experience a reduced quality of life: https://pubmed.ncbi.nlm.nih.gov/12131746/

The emotional impact of scoliosis can be different for those who choose a nonsurgical, non-watch-and-wait treatment approach.

Functional, patient-centered treatment programs, such as those offered by the Scoliosis Reduction Center, offer patients the chance to live in a different emotional landscape.

From my experience, hope is one of the greatest antidotes to the negative emotions that often accompany scoliosis. Under the traditional model of treatment, hope exists in the form of a small glimmer offered by the promise of successful spinal surgery. But under the chiropractic model, hope exists in the form of actual reductions in abnormal spinal curvatures. And there's a lot of it to be found.

The hope that can be found in a promising treatment plan serves as a buoy for patients who struggle with the emotional impact of scoliosis. However, if you've not yet begun treatment for your condition—or if you have yet to be diagnosed—there is quite a bit you can do right now to help stabilize your emotional state.

In the next chapter, I will discuss how you can address both your physical and emotional pain in ways that make you stronger and better able to experience the benefits of treatment.

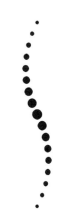

CHAPTER SEVEN

Will Anything Make the Pain Go Away?

THE PAIN ASSOCIATED WITH having scoliosis as an adult can be absolutely excruciating. The pain from adult scoliosis can make patients forget everything else and lose hope completely. Pain is such a powerful factor in the lives of adults with scoliosis that they'll do just about anything to experience some amount of relief.

Does this sound familiar?

I have a feeling that many readers of this book will skip directly to this chapter. From what I have seen in adults who have scoliosis, the desire to find effective pain relief is so strong that patients make it their mission to try anything that promises even a small amount of comfort. It's difficult for them to take a more holistic, structural perspective of their condition because they're often consumed by pain completely. It rules their lives, and their awareness tends to focus on the symptoms of pain and the relief that may be possible by treating those symptoms.

If you came to this chapter hoping to find some quick fixes for scoliosis pain, I'm afraid you may be disappointed. There are no secret tricks, tips, or hints that will make your pain go away. Relieving the pain of adult scoliosis isn't simple, and there are no quick fixes. So beware of anyone who tells you that their system or modality will relieve your pain without dealing with the structural realities of your scoliosis. It's just not true.

Does this mean that you'll have to endure your terrible scoliosis pain for the rest of your life? Not at all. It's possible to address and reduce your pain effectively—I see patients every day who have reduced their pain while improving mobility and function. You must keep in mind, though, that quick fixes and solutions that promise pain relief to be easy are usually not all that they're cracked up to be.

If you've been dealing with the pain of adult scoliosis for a while, you've probably tried a number of things to ease your pain. I've seen patients like you who have taken quite a journey through pain management only to end up with a more severe abnormal spinal curvature—and in a lot more pain. Sooner or later, it dawns on them that their pain isn't going to go away. Every time they do something to treat a symptom, the pain returns. Or they notice pain in other parts of the body.

In many cases, patients turn to pharmaceutical remedies like pain pills. Sadly, this can place individuals on a path that leads to dependence, addiction, illness, and sometimes even death. I can understand the allure of pain medications, and I get why patients are compelled to rely on them. They provide quick, significant relief. At least, at first, that's the case.

Patients who are prescribed pain pills can experience a remarkable amount of pain relief in the first days and weeks. They often regain physical abilities that had been dormant due to the presence of pain. They get some energy and vigor back. Spending time with friends and family is enjoyable again because they aren't preoccupied with pain.

As I'm sure you know, this relief rarely lasts. The body develops a tolerance for pain medications over time. This requires patients to take more pills just to feel the same effects. Physical dependence on these medications also complicates matters; after a while, the patient's dependence will become overwhelming. The pills no longer provide pain relief; they are necessary just to make the patient feel normal. It's a terrible cycle that can lead patients down some very dark roads.

The reason that pain pills don't work for scoliosis pain is that they focus on symptoms without addressing the underlying structural realities of the condition. As patients treat their pain points, the spine continues to progress into a greater abnormal curvature. This progression is the process that causes pain. Anything that fails to address it will fail to relieve the patient's pain. So although pain pills can provide real relief, any amount of comfort they bring is just a detour.

Even patients who have felt adamant about avoiding pain pills will sometimes succumb to them, given their ability to provide some amount of relief. In many cases, these patients will seek out more "natural" remedies. They will improve their diets by eating more whole foods that are free of processing and the presence of extra sugar, fat, or additives. This is a good thing. An improved diet can help you stave off inflammation, boost your mood, and help your body's systems work more efficiently. But it's not going to do anything to stop or slow down the progression of your spine's curvature.

Is That Pain in Your Gut Scoliosis?

People are often surprised when they learn about the various ways in which scoliosis can manifest in the body. As you know, the pain it causes in the body might appear in areas that are nowhere near your spine, or they seem to be completely unconnected to your scoliosis. This is why providers tend to treat symptoms first without exploring what is actually at the root of the issue.

Scoliosis affects the body so comprehensively sometimes that it can even influence your digestive system. Maybe you were aware that scoliosis could cause pain in far-flung areas of your body. But did you know it could also contribute to conditions like constipation, stomach cramping, irritable bowel syndrome (IBS), acid reflux, and heartburn? Surprising, isn't it?

But think of it this way: your digestive system is a complex arrangement of organs that work together to process nutrients and supply the energy to your body from the foods that you eat. So if you have a condition that affects these organs in any way, it can also influence their function.

The thing about the spine is that it is, in fact, connected to every system of the body. So if it seems impossible that your scoliosis could have something to do with discomfort in your stomach, consider that your spine is sort of like the messenger of the body. Your brain is the command center, where all of the processing happens. It's also where signals are sent from. Those signals travel down the spine as if it's an interstate highway. They exit the main highway to travel down peripheral nerves, which are like smaller state or county roads. Those nerves convey the signals to the body's organs, including those that are used for digestion.

An abnormally curved spine is like a twisty, bumpy road—it creates a higher degree of difficulty for travel. It is also far less efficient than a nice flat, straight path. Therefore, the signals that your brain sends aren't conveyed nearly as efficiently.

Scoliosis can have a significant impact on your digestive system in a structural sense as well.

Your internal organs all have their places and positions within your body. With a healthy spine, every organ is given its natural amount of space to operate. But when you have an abnormally curved spine, the organs must fit more awkwardly within your body. They must often force themselves to fit into cramped positions, which can cause pain, discomfort, or other complications.

Digestion is a highly physical, mechanical process of the body. Your digestive organs require room to operate properly and go through this process effectively. But if the spine causes you to favor one side of the body over the other, compression and contortion occurs. Normal digestion becomes challenging for your stomach and other organs. Your intestines can become pinched or blocked, which can lead to constipation.

So to answer the question "Is that pain in your gut scoliosis?" well, it might not be. But I would be pretty surprised if your spine's condition wasn't a major contributor.

Because your spine is so central to everything that happens in your body, it might be a good idea to consider it as the culprit whenever you experience pain, discomfort, irritability or other troubling symptoms, regardless of where they may be occurring. You can certainly treat your symptoms, which might give you some temporary relief. But until you address the structural issues of your spine, it's highly likely that you'll continue to experience aches, pains, and other maladies as your scoliosis progresses.

Sometimes, patients will add exercise and activity to a healthier diet, expecting that their pain will subside if they make their bodies more physically active. Again, I can understand the instinct to get into an exercise regimen as an adult with painful scoliosis. For most people, the aches and pains associated with aging can be reduced considerably by adopting a healthier diet and more active lifestyle. But for adults with scoliosis, things are just not that simple.

In general, being fit and participating in an exercise program is something I recommend for scoliosis patients. Fitness is something that's very important to my daily life. And I see it's a major contributor to not only my quality of life, but also the quality of life my patients experience. A person who is fit and healthy is better equipped to handle treatment and participate in scoliosis-specific exercises. Typically, physical fitness provides important benefits to factors like mood and overall energy levels too, which helps motivate patients and keeps them hopeful in their treatment.

Although physical fitness, like diet, is important, it's ultimately not going to stop the progression of your scoliosis. It seems counterintuitive sometimes: it is quite common for me to hear patients talk about the importance of building their core strength. Logically, it makes sense for patients that if they improve their core muscles, it will prevent their scoliosis curves from worsening. But that isn't the case.

While I applaud any patient's desire to proactively improve their body and boost their fitness, I must also educate them about the crucial differences between exercises designed for general fitness and those that are meant to stabilize scoliosis.

For one thing, general exercises typically don't address the postural muscles of the spine; instead, they focus on building mass and power, which isn't helpful for those with scoliosis.

Traditional exercises have been designed for symmetrical bodies, so they work the muscles in a balanced manner. Individuals with scoliosis, however, have bodies that are, by definition, asymmetrical. For exercises to be truly helpful, scoliosis patients need to have them tailored to their specific scoliosis patterns. The issue with activities such as resistance training, yoga, or aerobic training is that they are almost never tailored to people who have scoliosis.

Typical gym exercises can also be highly compressive to the spine. For people who have scoliosis, such compression can actually cause harm to the spine and increase pain. In reality, the compressive nature of these types of exercises increases the risk to scoliosis patients of making the condition worse.

Many patients will see no harm in performing general aerobics or going to yoga classes. These forms of exercise are generally seen as low impact. And for most people, there is very little chance of becoming injured or exacerbating a previous injury/condition. But for individuals with scoliosis, the potential for harm increases considerably from even the lowest-impact activities.

Yoga, for example, stretches and strengthens the muscles differently from the typical types of exercises you would do at the gym. But that doesn't make it appropriate for people who have adult scoliosis.

Yoga is performed in a symmetrical manner—each side of the body goes through an identical set of stretches designed to stretch the muscles equally. However, treating scoliosis effectively requires a more asymmetrical approach. With the spine out of its normal alignment, there's no symmetry to maintain. Instead, it's necessary to work one side of the body more than the other to account for the spine's curvature. And the sides that are worked on will differ from patient to patient, based on the area of the spine that's activated. Someone with an S curve, for example, may need to work the lumbar area of the spine on one side, while working the thoracic area of the other side. It requires a type of specificity that is almost never accounted for in most yoga practices.

There are "safe" forms of general exercise, like swimming or working out on the elliptical machine, that involve virtually no compression of the spine. That makes them good options for scoliosis patients who want to maintain or improve their general fitness. But even these safe forms of exercise do nothing to address the progression of scoliosis.

As you can see, even healthy activities like going to the gym or participating in yoga can have a harmful effect on adults with scoliosis. At best, "safe" exercises have no effect on the progression of scoliosis, though they may provide a boost in overall fitness. It can be heartbreaking, particularly for those who have wanted to take on the condition and treat it with sheer force of will. They believe that if they just do the right exercises and live the right lifestyle, they can defeat their scoliosis and return to a normal, pain-free life. Unfortunately, this never comes to pass. Meanwhile, the pain continues to grow stronger and spread to new areas of the body. They lose function. They feel their energy levels melt away. Eventually, even those who were ardently against taking pain pills succumb to their allure.

Surgery also becomes an increasingly appealing option for adults living with the pain of their scoliosis. Over time, they become convinced that limited mobility is a fair trade-off for the promise of pain relief. Unfortunately, pain relief is never guaranteed.

For people without scoliosis, undergoing an expensive, invasive spinal-fusion surgery is the last thing they would want to do. But for adults who have been living with scoliosis pain that only gets worse over time, surgery can hold quite a bit of promise. It's a trade-off, to be sure, but it is one that adults with scoliosis are often willing to live with. Even when told that surgery will alter their bodies irreversibly, cause complications and provide no guaranteed pain relief, adults with scoliosis will eagerly sign up for it. Why? Because it's a way out. It is a way out of pain and suffering. It's a way out of continuous progression. It is a way out of watching and waiting. It's the chance to have a new life.

To me, surgery should only be considered as an absolute last resort for treating adults with scoliosis. The dominant narrative about scoliosis in our society says that surgery is the natural end

EXPLORING ADULT SCOLIOSIS

point for the condition. But that's just not true. As I have written previously, I think surgery should be viewed not as an ending, but as a new beginning. Patients may no longer have to deal with certain issues related to their scoliosis, but they are only trading in those challenges for a set of new ones.

All the normal methods of treating pain are ultimately ineffective when it comes to scoliosis in adults. Natural methods and pharmaceutical methods are equally stymied by the condition. It can seem like there's nothing you can do.

Furthermore, the increasing physical pain you experience is accompanied by emotional challenges that add to the complexity of your suffering. Yes, you can treat the emotional pain directly, which may provide some relief. Things like visiting a therapist, practicing mindfulness, spending time with loved ones, taking care of another person (or pet) are all wonderful ways to ease your emotional strain. I recommend doing whatever natural, healthy activities you can to help your heart and head feel better as you cope with the pain of scoliosis.

But the source of much of your emotional pain is also the source of your physical pain if you're an adult who has scoliosis. Eventually, the abnormal curvature of your spine (and its progression) will need to be addressed in order to provide any kind of relief, physical, emotional or otherwise.

So, if all the usual methods of treating pain don't work for your scoliosis, what else is there?

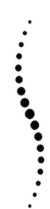

CHAPTER EIGHT

Imagine a Life without Scoliosis Pain—How Can You Get There?

WHEN I SEE PATIENTS overcome the pain of living with scoliosis as an adult, it gives me a great, positive feeling. I believe that we, as human beings, are here to live rich, fulfilling lives that aren't limited by conditions like scoliosis. But for adults like you who have such a painful condition, that kind of life just doesn't seem possible. It's just too hard to envision.

Here's my challenge to you: Picture your life free from the terrible pain of scoliosis. You're healthy, active, and smiling. Surrounded by loved ones, you are able to focus on your time with them instead of focusing on your body and how it feels. You notice that, for the first time in what seems like forever, you feel good in your body. Mornings are spent feeling well rested and excited about the day ahead. Evenings are spent relaxing and enjoying the fruits of your labors. In between, you're living your life and doing the things you want to do—all without being dominated by the pain of scoliosis.

Like so many adults who have scoliosis, picturing this type of scenario can be simultaneously hopeful and frustrating. It can be fun to escape into this type of fantasy and imagine it coming true. But it can also be devastating when you have to come back to earth and live with your current amount of pain. Here's the thing: Your vision of a life free from scoliosis pain doesn't have to be a fantasy. It can be reality. And you don't have to suffer through surgery to get there.

So, what's the catch?

There is no catch. You just have to be prepared for a new journey. It's not going to be an easy one, but it will be one of the most rewarding journeys of your life. It will require you to take on new challenges and endure treatments that may sometimes feel more challenging than the condition you're fighting. You may not like the path that leads you to a life free from so much pain, but it's the only way forward if you want to improve your life quality and potentially reduce your abnormal curvature without going through surgery.

The functional approach to treating scoliosis in adults may seem like an alternative to the standard methods that have been around for decades. But to me, methods like watching and waiting and surgery are completely outdated. The surgical approach to treating scoliosis should have been outmoded long ago in favor of methods that address the underlying structural issues. To me, it is only a valid option when used as a last resort. Unfortunately, the orthopedic model is too well established to budge from its position of prominence.

I believe that the chiropractic-focused approach to treating scoliosis will eventually become as common, accepted, and standardized as air travel. Consider what people used to say about the concept of aviation: they thought it would be impossible at worst or foolishly dangerous at best. Those people weren't wrong. For them, they had yet to see a well-designed aircraft that was capable of transporting people safely and efficiently through the air. So for decades, people considered the possibility of air travel as an out-there, fringe idea.

These days, the conventional wisdom says conservative scoliosis treatment is impossible. In my view, that is only because people haven't experienced a complete, comprehensive, and well-designed program. To them, it's impossible.

Things change, though. Today, everyone agrees that air travel is the safest, most efficient way to move across long distances. It might even be impossible for you to imagine life without it. The same is true for conservative treatment of adult scoliosis. You may believe that such treatment wouldn't be effective because you have seen no evidence to support it. And you're not wrong.

Part of my job is to show you that you don't have to wait for conservative treatment approaches to become legitimate—they are already helping patients live better lives and helping individuals like you avoid surgery. To me, chiropractic-focused scoliosis treatment is the new gold standard.

Aviation pioneers eventually made the airplane into the modern standard for travel; I hope this book will show you that my predecessors, colleagues, and I have made conservative treatment the model for addressing adult scoliosis the right way.

The things you believe play a huge role in your ability to treat scoliosis effectively. If you believe that conservative treatment won't help you, it probably won't, especially if you've seen no evidence or examples of its effectiveness. But if you believe in the power of chiropractic-focused treatment, you are more likely to buy in, commit to it, and see actual improvements.

Do you believe it is possible to live life as an adult without enduring so much pain? Do you believe that you can get there without going through surgery? Do you believe you have what it takes to fight your scoliosis using functional treatment? Do you believe you can reduce your abnormal curvature?

I believe in you too.

In the next sections of this book, I will help you explore in more detail what your life can look like. First, I will describe the consequences of staying on a path of inaction. Then I'll go deeper into the actions you can take to move forward in a way that puts you in charge of your scoliosis.

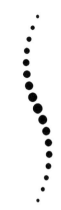

The Real Consequences of Life with Adult Scoliosis

WHAT IS THIS LIFE about for you?

Is it about taking action, or is it about waiting for something good to happen?

Whether you've had scoliosis since adolescence or have developed it in adulthood, the condition can make you feel as though you're not in charge. So you watch and wait because that is what the "experts" all seem to recommend.

You aren't powerless right now, but I understand if that is how you feel, especially considering the dominant narratives about scoliosis in our society.

In this section, I will explore what your life will look like if you take on watching and waiting as your strategy. I'll warn you now that it isn't a pretty picture. However, I believe it's important to paint this picture so you and other adults with scoliosis understand what's in store if you continue down the path of inaction.

Don't worry. This section may be a little sobering, but it's not all doom and gloom. In my life and in my practice at the Scoliosis

Reduction Center, I'm a big believer in the power of hope. So keep in mind that nothing I describe about the challenges of living with scoliosis is set in stone. If you take action and opt to treat your scoliosis functionally and proactively, you can write an entirely different story for yourself.

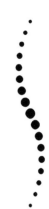

CHAPTER NINE

A Life of Limitation and Pain Management

WHAT ARE THE THINGS you like to do in life?

Like many adults, you're probably devoted to your children and family. There is a transformation that happens in adulthood when people become far less self-centered than they were in their younger years. The well-being of others takes on new significance, especially for those who have taken on the responsibility of starting and raising a family.

It is common for adults with scoliosis to allow their condition to progress in the background as they live through their twenties and thirties. It's a busy, beautiful time of life, and it's often characterized by the act of building a family. Those me-first instincts of youth have receded in favor of instincts that benefit the family unit you are a part of. Younger adults with scoliosis may also be experiencing quite mild symptoms at this point in their lives, making the condition seem much less urgent.

Another transformation happens in adulthood once children have been raised and have begun to live their own independent lives. For a lot of adults, the possibility of new beginnings opens up to them in their thirties, forties, and fifties. The kids are off to college, and it's time to take stock of what's possible now.

Faced with newfound freedom, adults at this stage in life can do some amazing things. They can continue to mentor and nurture their children with wisdom and advice. But they have more time and energy at this stage than ever before to pursue their true passions.

This is a vibrant time of life for adults. It's a time to develop new skills, learn more about the world, and be an active participant in the world.

For adults with scoliosis, however, this is a time of life that can feel lonesome, exhausting, and painful.

Whatever you like to do with your life, or whatever your plans are for your future, scoliosis has a way of putting up stop signs and routing you through tedious detours on a road you should be thoroughly enjoying.

Beware These Scoliosis Myths

Scoliosis is an interesting condition for a number of reasons. The fact that most cases have no known cause (i.e., are "idiopathic") often throws people for a loop. Its progressive nature also gives it different characteristics as a person with the condition ages. So not only does it manifest differently from patient to patient; it can manifest differently in the *same* patient as it progresses over time.

From my perspective, it seems like members of the general public have a basic awareness of scoliosis as a condition of the spine. But beyond that, understanding of the condition is cloudy, at best, and just plain wrong, at worst. In other words, a lot of people know that there's a condition of the spine called *scoliosis*, but if you go beneath the surface of their understanding, you'll find quite a bit of myth and misinformation.

Unfortunately, there are numerous scoliosis myths that are taken as fact, even today when actual facts about the condition are easy to find. I feel that these myths are worth calling out because they aren't just harmless pieces of misinformation; rather, they are potentially quite harmful to adults like you who have the condition and want to do something about it.

These persistent myths can be debunked fairly easily, but that doesn't mean they'll go away. Although I have been writing and speaking about them for years now, I'm often surprised by how powerful they continue to be in the minds of people who, frankly, should know better.

The fact is that widespread belief in these scoliosis myths leads to real suffering. When these myths are allowed to be seen as truth, they muddy the waters of understanding and prevent people from taking action that can actually restore function and reduce abnormal spinal curvatures.

Myth #1—Your Progression and Pain Will Go Away on Their Own

If I could change one thing about the general perception of adult scoliosis, it's this. There is still much to learn about the nature of scoliosis, but one thing we know for sure, without a doubt, is that scoliosis progresses over time. The progression may be barely perceptible, or it may be significant, but it always happens.

As scoliosis progresses—and, let me repeat, it *always* progresses— the pain associated with the condition never improves; it only worsens over time.

If you have a mild curvature right now and experience very little to no pain, you might feel like you're out of the woods, with regard to how your scoliosis will impact your life. The truth is that your journey with the condition is only beginning. Your scoliosis will become increasingly severe over time, leading to more and more complications and challenges. Pain will increase in severity and duration. Sooner or later, you'll need to take action. But why let it get to that point? Why not take action now? Treating your scoliosis now when it's still mild may seem like overkill, but being proactive with the condition is always preferable to watching and waiting. Always.

I have seen patients on the other end of the pain spectrum who continue to hold on to the mistaken belief that their pain will disappear on its own somehow. They live their lives in severe discomfort. Scoliosis literally dominates their days. And yet, they believe that if they just wait it out, their bodies will adjust, the progression of the condition will stop, and they will be able to go on living pain-free.

Not true.

No matter what stage of scoliosis you are experiencing right now, it will be more severe tomorrow. Your pain will increase steadily over time as your abnormal curvature progresses. You don't have to let it be this way, though.

This myth is incredibly powerful and persuasive. The allure of having a condition go away on its own without intervention is enough to keep people from seeking treatment. This leaves people living in pain and discomfort, often watching and waiting until they get the go-ahead to have spinal-fusion surgery.

You can do better.

Myth #2—The Progression of Your Curvature Can Be Predicted Reliably

If you've been living with scoliosis for most of your life, you might be under the impression that your scoliosis will progress at the same rate it has always progressed. It can feel like scoliosis is such a well-known part of yourself that you have an innate "knowing" about what it will do next.

The truth is that there is no telling how your scoliosis curvature will progress in the future. While it may certainly continue progressing at the rate you've become accustomed to, that is unlikely. Typically, the larger the curve becomes, the quicker the rate of progression increases. The rate of progression also increases as patients grow older. In all likelihood, these two factors will ensure that the rate of your curvature's progression will only increase the longer you wait.

Again, you may think you have a handle on adult scoliosis, but the condition will always be progressing in the background, on its own terms and at its own speed. This is yet another reason why taking early action is preferable to watching and waiting.

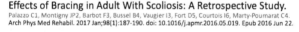

Effects of Bracing in Adult With Scoliosis: A Retrospective Study.
Palazzo C1, Montigny JP2, Barbot F3, Bussel B4, Vaugier I3, Fort D5, Courtois I6, Marty-Poumarat C4.
Arch Phys Med Rehabil. 2017 Jan;98(1):187-190. doi: 10.1016/j.apmr.2016.05.019. Epub 2016 Jun 22.

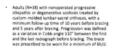

- Adults (N=38) with nonoperated progressive idiopathic or degenerative scoliosis treated by custom-molded lumbar-sacral orthoses, with a minimum follow-up time of 10 years before bracing and 5 years after bracing. Progression was defined as a variation in Cobb angle ≥10° between the first and the last radiograph before bracing. The brace was prescribed to be worn for a minimum of 6h/d.

- **RESULTS:**

- At the moment of bracing, the mean age was 61.3±8.2 years, and the mean Cobb angle was 49.6°±17.7°.

- For both types of scoliosis, the rate of progression decreased from 1.28°±.79°/y before to .21°±.43°/y after bracing (P<.0001).

- For degenerative scoliosis, it dropped from 1.47°±.83°/y before to .24°±.43°/y after bracing (P<.0001)

- Idiopathic dropped from .70°±.06°/y before to .24°±.43°/y after bracing (P=.03), respectively.

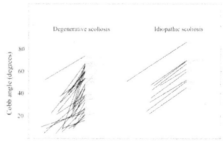

The truth is that every single adult patient I've worked with who has documentation of their curve going back twenty years can attest to the worsening of their curvature over time. Take a look at the graphic above for an example of how curvatures progress before treatment (the dark-black line) versus after treatment (the light-gray line). Clearly, you can see that pretreatment progression tends to be quite steady, increasing at a reliable rate over time. However, treatment halts this steady progress—often reversing it. This is a great illustration of the differences between watching and waiting versus taking action to treat the condition functionally.

Myth #3—The Best Way to Fix Scoliosis Is Spinal-Fusion Surgery

This, sadly, is the dominant narrative about treating scoliosis. If you ask the average person how scoliosis is treated most effectively, they will probably mention surgery. This false idea is so deeply ingrained in our collective consciousness that people rarely consider that there may be alternatives. Surgery is seen as an ending; it's seen as a "fix." The fact is that surgery isn't a fix for the condition at all. It's just the mark of a new beginning.

The reason this mindset dominates is that traditional conservative treatments of scoliosis are just not effective. Therefore, doctors who are unaware of alternative treatments or the chiropractic-centered approach conclude that surgery is the only way forward.

Surgery can stabilize scoliosis, but it isn't a cure. Complications can arise from surgery that introduce a whole new host of problems into the body. And having one surgery is no guarantee that another won't be necessary a few years down the road.

Going into surgery represents the traditional method of dealing with scoliosis. It's the most well-known method, and it's one that countless people with scoliosis have sought for treatment. But it isn't the best way to treat scoliosis.

The best way to treat scoliosis is address it directly, from a functional perspective. Those who have the condition don't have to watch and wait until it's time for surgery. They can put in the work to reduce their curvatures, regain function, and reduce their pain levels. While doing this, they transform surgery from an inevitability to an absolute last resort. And that's exactly how it should be.

Myth #4—Scoliosis Is Only a Problem if Your Doctor Says So

This is a very commonly accepted myth, and one that causes a lot of frustration.

Doctors who operate in the traditional health-care model don't always understand scoliosis and are often reluctant to acknowledge that it even exists in a patient's spine. Generally, they view health issues through the lens of the tools they have to fix them. For most doctors, their most powerful tool is surgery, so if surgery is deemed inappropriate for the issue, then it must not be an issue.

What happens is that doctors will talk about all the issues caused by the abnormal curvature of the spine without ever addressing the underlying condition. They'll mention conditions like arthritis, spinal stenosis, herniations, and so on—the list goes on and on. They will offer treatments and solutions for these secondary conditions, none of which work long term, because they fail to address the real issue that's causing the conditions.

Eventually, doctors will concede that scoliosis is the issue that must be addressed. But they will only do so once the condition has become severe, requiring surgery.

My advice is to trust your gut. If you suspect that your scoliosis is causing secondary health conditions, but your doctor won't acknowledge it, it's probably only a matter of time before the condition becomes so severe that surgery will be framed as your only choice going forward. If your concerns about scoliosis aren't being validated by your doctor, I would suggest seeking the advice of someone who actually specializes in scoliosis.

Watching your peers live active, fulfilling lives should be joyful and inspiring. But if you're living with scoliosis in adulthood, seeing what others your age can do with their lives may not make you feel so great. Seeing other people experiencing the world while you live with limitations and pain can make you feel like life has played a cruel trick on you.

Living a limited life can make you feel like you don't belong. Like there is something wrong with you. In my world, we talk frequently about how scoliosis can have negative impacts on the social lives of teenagers, but the impacts on adults can be just as painful. Your peers, knowing that you experience pain on a regular basis, may begin to not include you in gatherings or outings. They do it out of love and concern for you, of course, but inside, it can feel like you are being rejected.

Pain and limitation. These are the factors that characterize life with adult scoliosis. They're bad enough on their own, but when they work together, they can make life absolutely miserable. These factors also seem to compound and grow exponentially over time.

The presence of physical pain places limitations on what you can do with your life and what you can handle in social settings. This adds stress and anxiety to the mix, both of which contribute greatly to the emotional pain of scoliosis. Naturally, the emotional pain feeds into the physical pain, and vice versa. Which creates even more limitations.

This is your life. It's yours to live, and you should be the one to decide what your next moves are. But scoliosis has a way of stepping in saying you can't do what you want to do. So, do you surrender? Or are you going to take action?

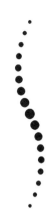

CHAPTER TEN

What Can You Expect if You Do Nothing about Your Scoliosis?

LIKE MOST OF US, you've probably envisioned a long, healthy life. Retirement spent traveling and hanging out with the grand-kids. New adventures over forty. Limitless possibilities. Full enjoyment. Sounds good, right?

Well, here's a particularly sobering statistic: According to a study detailed in *The Journal of Bone and Joint Surgery* (https://journals.lww.com/jbjsjournal/Citation/1971/53040/THE_ORTHOPAEDIC_RESEARCH_SOCIETY_.23.aspx), individuals who avoided treatment for their idiopathic scoliosis had their life expectancies reduced by as much as fourteen years. The study also indicated a 15 percent mortality rate.

The reality of life with adult scoliosis isn't one many people would spend time fantasizing about.

Just like the condition itself, your life with scoliosis will grow progressively worse over time. The visions you have of a new chapter for your life will become cloudier and less detailed. They may disappear entirely only to be replaced by darker visions of a painful future.

I can understand the appeal of doing nothing. In the short term, ignoring a problem is much easier than dealing with it head-on. And what if ignoring it actually works? Won't you feel silly having spent so much time and energy on a problem that would have solved itself if you had just left it alone?

Doing nothing is far more attractive than having spinal-fusion surgery. But here's the thing: spinal-fusion surgery is the final destination on the road of doing nothing. Under the traditional treatment model, the whole point is to have patients wait and watch their condition progress. Time is spent undergoing regular examinations and measurements until the point at which the spine's curvature has progressed to where surgery is recommended. It isn't an efficient system of treatment, nor is it effective. But it is the system that dominates conventional wisdom about how to treat scoliosis.

I cannot overstate the fact that surgery should never be seen as a quick fix. If you opt to undergo surgery, I have nothing but hope and kind wishes for you and your recovery. But the fact is that surgery increases the probability that you'll experience additional health issues. There is always a risk, and it should not be taken lightly.

It's likely that you will have a wide range of "experts" telling you that the smart thing to do with your adult scoliosis is to watch and wait. It is better to remain cautious and conservative, they might tell you, than it's to take action. But what's so cautious and conservative about putting patients on a one-way road to the operating table?

Real conservative treatment of scoliosis doesn't involve surgery. Rather, it involves a combination of treatment techniques designed specifically for each individual patient. The goal of this type of treatment is, in fact, to avoid surgery. So if caution and conservatism are important to you with regard to your treatment, doing nothing is actually counterintuitive.

How Does Scoliosis Affect the Elderly?

Scoliosis in adolescence should be treated as a serious condition, and it should be addressed as soon as possible. But it rarely causes pain or severe discomfort. There is also much more progression to occur in the future when it comes to the typical spine of a teen who has scoliosis.

In adulthood, scoliosis becomes painful. To the point where the lives that patients live can be affected quite adversely. Not only is it painful, it has progressed since adolescence if the patient has been living with adolescent idiopathic scoliosis (AIS), so it is likely to cause additional challenges and complications.

But what about scoliosis in the elderly?

I'm sure you can guess that it never improves in one's golden years. It only continues its progression, leading to increased pain and an even greater number of troubling complications.

Scoliosis is actually quite common among the elderly, too. Among individuals over the age of sixty-five who have *no* low back pain, scoliosis was found to exist in 68 percent of study participants. Just imagine if the study had included those who experience back pain. The number would likely be much higher.

If you think about it, the high prevalence of scoliosis among the elderly makes perfect sense: People who had mild or nonexistent scoliosis in their adolescence or adulthood grew into elderly individuals. All the while as they aged, their scoliosis continued to progress into their geriatric years. Others developed degenerative—or De

Novo—scoliosis at some point in adulthood. Again, this type of scoliosis is progressive, so by the time a patient reaches retirement age, it can become severe.

There is also the type of scoliosis that can happen from trauma, after a severe injury or surgery.

By the time a person has reached advanced age, there's ample opportunity for scoliosis to arrive, develop and become a very serious condition. And at this time, the only procedure that's recommended under the traditional model of treatment is surgery.

Surgery is risky in patients at any age. But for elderly patients, the risk is considerably higher. What's more, recovery from surgery tends to take much longer and the possibility of complications arising becomes greater as well. Successful surgery for an elderly person isn't the end of the road, either. For older patients, there is an increased chance that they will require additional "revision" surgeries further down the road.

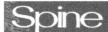

Short-term mortality and its association with independent risk factors in adult spinal deformity surgery.

Pateder DB[1], Gonzales RA, Kebaish KM, Cohen DB, Chang JY, Kostuik JP

⊕ Author Information

Abstract
STUDY DESIGN: Retrospective review

OBJECTIVES: To determine postoperative mortality after adult spinal deformity surgery. To determine whether independent risk factors can predict mortality

SUMMARY OF BACKGROUND DATA: Although mortality after adult spinal surgery is reported to range from 0.03% to 3.52%, there is a general paucity of data on mortality and its associated risk factors after adult spinal deformity surgery.

METHODS: Three hundred sixty-one adults with spinal deformity underwent 407 corrective procedures. For patients who died within 30 days of the procedure, the following risk factors were examined to determine if each could independently predict mortality: demographic information, American Society of Anesthesiologists' (ASA) classification; operative time, surgical approach, number of fusion levels, primary versus revision surgery, and intraoperative blood loss.

RESULTS: Ten of the 407 procedures resulted in death (2.4% mortality): 1 intraoperatively secondary to cardiac ischemia, 3 secondary to sepsis/multiple organ failure, 2 each secondary to pulmonary embolus, uncal herniation/cerebral edema, and shock. The average preoperative ASA levels for patients who died and patients who survived were 3.0 and 2.3, respectively (P < 0.0001). Age, gender, operative time, surgical approach, number of fusion levels, revision status, and estimated blood loss did not have an independently significant correlation to mortality.

CONCLUSION: There was a strong association (P < 0.0001) between increasing ASA class and increasing mortality. The other risk factors could not independently predict postoperative mortality within 30 days after adult spinal deformity surgery.

Take a look at this study, which focused on the mortality rates of patients after undergoing scoliosis surgery. Patients were followed for just thirty days after their procedures, revealing a death rate of 2.4 percent, which is alarming. Imagine if the study followed people for two years, postsurgery. I have no doubt that the rate would rise to an even more alarming number.

Elderly patients with scoliosis should never assume that surgery is their best option. The fact is that surgery cannot "fix" scoliosis, certainly not for the duration of the patient's life. And when surgeries fail to produce the desired results, there's usually no other option presented beyond additional surgeries.

A functional, nonsurgical, patient-centered approach to treating scoliosis can be effective for elderly patients, but it's also preferable to treat patients as early as possible. Trust me—you don't want to wait until you've reached retirement age or older to start treating your scoliosis. So if you think you can wait, even if it's just another year, don't. Those years have a way of stacking up quickly in adulthood. Before you know it, you may be in excruciating pain, living a limited life in what should be a time of enjoyment.

Let's say you stay on the path of watching and waiting. How will your life unfold?

For one thing, the pain that has come to define your days will only increase. While you may have good days and bad days, the bad days will grow progressively worse as the good ones become fewer and farther in between. What's more, the places where pain exists in your body will grow in number, and those areas will spread in size. Eventually, there may be more areas of your body that are in pain than those that are not.

With increased pain will come a decrease in your ability to do the things you love. As your body takes on increasing pain, your mind will become devoted to thinking about your pain and how to soothe it. This will make you unable to participate fully in conversations or social gatherings. Your ability to be present and focused in such situations will decline because you will become preoccupied with pain and pain management.

Eventually, the pain and discomfort from your condition will overtake you and assume control of your life. This won't happen overnight, either, which makes it quite insidious. Slowly, your body will surrender, little by little, to the realities of your condition and the pain it causes. Your life will become all about managing pain, keeping your energy levels up and trying to get good sleep.

Emotionally and mentally, scoliosis will take a huge toll. As if the physical pain of scoliosis were not enough, the mental resources you would normally rely on are given over to dealing with your pain and discomfort. Your energy becomes scarce, and your mood begins to darken. People see a smile on your face less and less. The sound of laughter diminishes. Your social circle tightens and thins.

At this point, surgery might seem like a miracle. You would do anything to relieve your pain and regain your life, even if it means spending a fortune and undergoing a procedure that may introduce more problems than it solves. Where once you thought you were being cautious with your condition, now you have become willing to undergo potentially risky spinal-fusion surgery.

This isn't a pretty picture, is it? The future you who does nothing with your scoliosis is probably an unhappy, unfulfilled person in a lot of pain, both physically and emotionally. This future version of yourself has drifted so far from your core values that surgery has become the most reasonable available option. The sad thing is that many people just like you are told that this is the best they can do.

Take a moment to go back to the vision of your life that I suggested at the beginning of this chapter. The grandchildren. The travel. The limitless possibilities. The freedom. Is this life possible if you do nothing about your scoliosis? I suppose it can't be ruled out. However, a life like this is pretty unlikely, given the progressive nature of your condition.

Hope is always available, no matter where you are on your scoliosis journey. But hope requires action to stay alive. The do-nothing, watch-and-wait approach to scoliosis treatment keeps you on the sidelines—and it's the surest way to deplete the hope you have for your future.

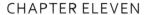

CHAPTER ELEVEN

One Person at the Beginning of the Day; Another Person at Night

FOR MANY PEOPLE WITH scoliosis in adulthood, the strange experience of going to bed as one person and waking up as another is pretty common.

If you're like others with your condition, this might sound familiar:

- Morning you wakes up feeling energized, refreshed and relatively free from pain.
- Evening you goes to bed feeling exhausted, irritated and filled with intense pain.

- Morning you gets out of bed with big plans for the day (and lots of time to get things done).
- Evening you gets into bed wondering where the day went (and how it went so quickly).

- Morning you focuses on coffee, breakfast and getting to work.
- Evening you focus on pain and discomfort.

- Morning you feels like life is full of possibilities.
- Evening you feels completely defeated by scoliosis.

I could go on, but I bet you get the picture.

This is a familiar cycle for many adults who live with scoliosis. Hope-filled mornings give way eventually to evenings filled with pain. Every morning, you wake up feeling better than you did the night before. But if you pay close attention, you'll notice that the relief you feel in the morning dwindles a little bit each day.

When adults with scoliosis feel good in the morning, their optimism can convince them that the condition might actually be getting better. So they put off making appointments or doing research into effective treatments. They think that because it feels good now, it might feel even better later. This optimism is almost always misguided.

When you feel at your worst, all you want to do is lie down and go to sleep. You don't have the energy to pursue treatments, make phone calls, or talk to those who might be able to help. But in the morning when you have the energy to take action, the reduction in pain and discomfort gives you just enough optimism to put off those actions for another day. And the cycle continues.

How to Get a Better Night's Sleep with Scoliosis

As an adult with scoliosis, getting a good night of sleep can mean the difference between having a good day and having it turn into a disaster. When you feel good in the morning, it's because you've taken the compressive load off of your body and spine for several hours, but it is also due to the healing, restorative power of sleep.

Although you may feel powerless to do anything about your scoliosis, you can gain an edge by maximizing the quality and amount of sleep you get.

Here are some tips:

- **Watch what you put into your body**—Your diet has a profound impact on your sleep patterns. Eating spicy, sugary, fatty, or overly processed foods will likely hamper your ability to get good sleep. Drinking alcohol is also a no-no: Even though its intoxication will help you get to sleep, the quality and duration of your sleep will be reduced considerably. You should also avoid eating in the hour or two prior to bedtime, which can limit your body's ability to transition into rest. Overall, you should try to consume more whole foods, fruits, and vegetables. Although a healthy diet isn't an effective treatment for scoliosis on its own, it's a critical aspect of giving the body what it needs to be as flexible and free from inflammation as possible.

- **Create a sanctuary for sleep**—How would you describe your bedroom? Is it a cluttered mess with a bed in the middle of it? Or is it a calming oasis where you can feel your most relaxed? Getting a good night's sleep is a lot easier when you love the room you're sleeping in. Your bedroom should be inviting, featuring light and decoration that makes you feel at ease and ready to transition into dreamtime. Waking up in a pleasant environment also adds to your overall sense of well-being, so it definitely pays to turn your sleeping space into a sanctuary.

- **Develop a sleep routine**—I know many adults who have never developed a nighttime routine. Their sleep is erratic, and their moods can be all over the place. Some of these people don't even have scoliosis. But in all seriousness, a routine at night can bring a significant amount of stability to your life. There should be a conscious "powering down" at night, which means taking steps that put you in a relaxed, calm state before resting your head on the pillow. Turn down the lights. Do some reading. Practice breathing exercises or meditation. It's really up to you how your routine will look. Whatever you do, though, your electronic devices (including your phone.) should not be included in your sleep routine. Staring at a screen in the hour or so leading up to bedtime can seriously disrupt your ability to get to sleep.

- **Find the right sleeping position**—While sleeping, your back should be supported and aligned. Your body should feel comfortable and not strained. The specific position that works best for you will be different from what works for another person. However, you should always avoid sleeping on your stomach. Sleeping on your stomach forces you to turn your head, which twists your spine and puts it out of alignment. Another bit of advice is to sleep in such a way that gravity pushes your curvature in the opposite direction. So if your curve goes to the right, for example, sleeping on your left side might allow you to put less strain on your body, giving you a better chance to have a good night of sleep.

Sleep is so critical that we give each patient at the Scoliosis Reduction Center a comprehensive sleep-routine plan. Essentially, it prepares the spine for a restful, restorative and healing night of sleep. It includes simple exercises and stretches as well as visualization practices, all of which are designed for each individual patient and their specific curve type. The routine is meant to work in a corrective fashion, helping the spine to maximize its healing potential while sleeping.

This dichotomy of being one person in the morning and another at night can feel like a real-life Dr. Jekyll and Mr. Hyde scenario. Except it is far from entertaining for the person who is living through it. In fact, it's downright terrible.

The ways to escape this scenario aren't always obvious. You can try to get better sleep, which can help bring you some relief.

But that isn't stopping the cycle; it's just making it slightly easier to endure. You can turn to pain pills, sedatives and other pharmaceutical methods to soften the impact of your pain and discomfort, but doing so only brings temporary relief while your scoliosis continues to progress inside your body. You can hope to become a candidate for surgery, but that is the last thing you should be doing in your quest for relief.

This cycle comes on slowly. You might be living inside it and not even know it. For many adults with scoliosis, recognizing this reality only happens after their condition has reached extremely painful levels. And they think it's too late to act.

Although the cycle I'm describing is familiar to adults like you with scoliosis, it isn't some rite of passage you are required to go through. You don't have to go to bed feeling awful. You don't have to let the promise of the day's beginning fade away into disappointment as the hours pass by and your pain increases.

Sometimes, there are exceptions to the way this cycle plays out, but they're equally unpleasant, if not more so. One exception is when the spine's curvature progresses to the point that it causes nerve pain, numbness, or radiculopathy, or some combination of these. These types of pains increase in their intensity after sleeping, causing patients to feel worse than when they fell asleep. Patients experiencing this scenario must try to fall asleep without focusing on the pain and how it will likely be worse when they wake up. This creates an entirely different cycle that leaves patients often experiencing a severe lack of sleep.

Another possible scenario occurs when patients with scoliosis develop issues in their extremities (typically in the lower portion of the body, commonly affecting hips and knees). Lying down to sleep can create relief and a reduction in pain. Unfortunately, getting up and putting a load on the joints brings the pain right back.

You can, in fact, go to bed at night feeling just as amazing as you did when you woke up in the morning. But it's not going to happen without you taking action. Scoliosis never gets better on its own.

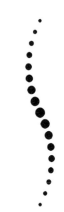

CHAPTER TWELVE

It's Never Going to Get Better on Its Own

YOU HAVE GOOD DAYS. You have bad days.

You have mornings of hope. You have evenings of pain. Back and forth, over and over. It's like a malfunctioning carnival ride with no exit and no way to take control.

Having scoliosis as an adult often means suffering. So much of your life is characterized by pain and discomfort that the small glimpses of relief you feel every once in a while seem to hold much more promise than is actually possible.

All you want is to feel better. To regain some function. To not worry about how your scoliosis affects things like your appearance or your social life. To not live in near-constant pain. So on those rare occasions when you wake up feeling like a million dollars, you feel like maybe you got over the hump. It can feel like the possibility of a new life is right there for the taking.

Inevitably, the pain will return. If not later that day, then sometime very soon. You think, *Tomorrow, I'll take action. Tomorrow, I'll make that appointment. Tomorrow...* But then you wake up feeling great again, so you decline to take action. Days, weeks, months, and years pass. Do you feel any better? Have you regained function? Has your life improved in any meaningful ways?

It's important to me that adults with scoliosis feel hope around their condition. Sadly, all too often, I see adults with the condition fill themselves with false hope based on the fact that they had one good day. Now, telling you that scoliosis will never get better on its own might seem like a hopeless message, but it's really a liberating one.

Living in the mistaken belief that scoliosis will improve on its own might allow a person to feel some amount of hope. That hope dwindles, though, because the condition just keeps on progressing relentlessly with decreasing evidence that it will ever stabilize or improve on its own.

In my opinion, hope comes from acceptance of reality. And if you're an adult who is living with scoliosis, the reality is that your condition will only worsen if you do nothing. Maybe one day you will become a candidate for spinal-fusion surgery, but that's nothing to be hopeful about.

Accepting this reality doesn't mean closing the door on hope. Rather, it opens up a whole new set of doors. When you accept the reality about scoliosis, you realize that you do, in fact, have a say in how it will affect you and the rest of your life. With you in charge of your body, your scoliosis and your life, you become empowered to make choices instead of waiting for them to be made for you. This can create a flood of hopeful feelings, which in turn create a boost in an adult patient's ability to seek treatment and stick with the program that will work for them, individually.

What's So Wrong with Observation?

Already in this book, you've seen it mentioned a number of times: Watch and wait, or wait and see. Under the traditional model of scoliosis treatment, this approach is also referred to as *observation*.

Observation—it sounds serious, cautious, and reasonable. It's a word used a lot by people in the realm of "experts." And it's used to explain all the reasons why you need to wait before you should address the structural issues of your spine.

But in reality, when doctors and others in the traditional model of treatment use the word *observation*, what they are referring to is doing nothing at all.

Maybe that sounds harsh, but that's the way scoliosis is treated under the established medical model. Conventional wisdom says that this is the best approach. Keeping an eye on the condition, it's believed, allows patients and doctors to make the best choices. I simply don't agree.

When you consider the type of treatment you would like to have for your scoliosis, you probably don't think, *I want to have the most mediocre and moderately effective treatment available.* No, you think that you should pursue the best-possible treatment plan, right? You want to see doctors and other specialists who understand the condition with modern, up-to-date perspectives. You want to involve yourself in a system that cares about you and your ability to live your best life. You deserve the best-possible treatment.

The only thing is that there is a significant difference of opinion among scoliosis experts when it comes to what the best-possible treatment entails.

In researching the best treatments available, you have probably come across the observation method, also known as *watch and wait.* It's often presented as the most reasonable path forward for people like you who have scoliosis in adulthood. But again, it's a method of treatment that involves nothing more than making observations of your condition from time to time. There's no action.

The truth about observation is that it's never the most effective approach for treating scoliosis, regardless of your age or the severity of your condition.

This approach is founded on the belief that surgery is the most effective treatment for scoliosis. At one time, there was very little evidence to support the efficacy of functional treatment or chiropractic-focused treatment of scoliosis. Not long ago, surgery was the only game in town. So doctors learned that watching and waiting was the best course of action. It was thought that surgery should only be performed once a patient's scoliosis curvature reached a certain severity level, typically forty degrees or more. Therefore, all doctors and patients could do was observe until which point the risk of surgery became an option.

The fact is that we have many more options for treatment available today. The conventional wisdom around treating scoliosis has shifted considerably. Now, more and more people are aware of functional-treatment options and the fact that abnormal spinal curvatures can actually be reduced. There is quite a bit of evidence to support the effectiveness of conservative, functional treatment too, unlike there had been in the past.

So, if your doctor is recommending observation on the way to eventual surgery, does that mean they are knowingly putting you on the wrong path?

No. Again, most doctors who treat scoliosis under the traditional model truly believe that their approach is the best. They are only following established medical principles, and they probably have your best interests in mind. Truly.

Also, if you were a spinal surgeon, you would see the world through a spinal surgeon's eyes. It's a perspective that holds surgery in high regard, as you would imagine. Have you heard the adage that if your only tool is a hammer, you'll see every problem as a nail? It's kind of like that when it comes to providers who operate under the traditional model of treatment. You can't blame them for simply doing what their profession says is best.

However, you don't have to take their word for it that their way is the best way, especially if you have the knowledge about nonsurgical treatments on your side. I would advise that if you have been given the advice to watch and wait, wait and see, or simply observe, you should continue your search for the most effective—and best— treatment for you.

The fact that scoliosis will never improve on its own is well known to experts and providers in the field. There is actually no debate around the topic of whether scoliosis is progressive in adults or not; it simply is a progressive condition. Full stop. Even those providers who recommend observation or the watch-and-wait approach understand that a patient's curvature will progress over time. It's just not a controversial subject.

I must admit that there are extremely rare cases of scoliosis in adults that reach a certain level and then stop progressing. So, is it technically possible that your curvature will discontinue its progression at some point? Sure, technically, that's possible. But it's highly improbable. You can never know if or when your progression will discontinue, so is that a risk you're willing to take?

Even if your curve stopped progressing, though, it would remain abnormal for the rest of your life, causing continuously challenging health issues as you grow older. Perhaps you could avoid surgery under this scenario, which would be great, but you would still have to live the rest of your life experiencing troubling—and potentially quite painful—symptoms.

So why is the path of inaction so popular?

It's the status quo. It's the established model. It's the king of the hill. It can be difficult for people to adopt new ways of thinking about certain subjects when established thought models have been so deeply entrenched in our thinking. Under the traditional model, there's nothing hopeful to offer patients, so inaction is seen as the best that can be done. Even when there's a great deal of evidence to support the efficacy of nonsurgical treatments for scoliosis, established treatment models hold a considerable amount of power, simply because they've been around for such a long time.

The realities of life with adult scoliosis are normal to you by now, I'm sure.

Think about your younger self for a minute, though. Whether you had idiopathic scoliosis as a teen and it continued into adulthood, or if you developed scoliosis as an adult, the younger version of you was probably in a lot less pain than you are now.

Would that younger version of yourself tolerate the painful reality you're living in today? Would they simply accept that you're doing your best by doing nothing at all? Would they find it reasonable for you to look forward to surgery as the solution for your condition?

No. Your younger self would probably scream at you to do something about your scoliosis. At this point in your life, the condition has progressed over so much time that you're accustomed to it in many ways. But if you went from feeling good directly into feeling the way you do today, it would feel completely unfair.

Your life holds just as much promise today as it did when you were a teenager. The possibilities for your life are truly limitless, even if you're at the age when you're sending kids off to college or holding your grandchildren for the first time. You can do something about your scoliosis that doesn't involve watching, waiting, living in pain for decades or undergoing expensive, invasive surgery. And you can start doing it now.

Why should you take action? Well, why would you consciously choose to continue suffering? You can do this for yourself, and the chances that you will feel better are pretty high. If taking action on your own behalf isn't inspiring enough, then do it for the people in your life who love you.

Your children and the members of your family want to know you at your best. They want to hear your laughter and see your smiling face. They respect you and know that you have a lot to teach them about the world, through the stories you tell about your past and the example you set with your life as it is now.

Do you want to take action and start feeling better about your scoliosis? In the next section, I'll take you on a journey through the next stage of your life—the stage when you finally do something about your scoliosis.

Can You Do Something about Your Adult Scoliosis?

PAIN, SUFFERING, AND ENDLESS limitations. Perhaps you have felt resigned to a life that would be characterized by the effects of your condition. I know that many adults with scoliosis feel hopeless when it comes to the idea that they might actually improve their condition. In reality, adults just like you've had tremendous success treating their scoliosis without having to go under the knife for expensive, invasive surgery.

In this section, I'll provide a contrast to the previous one. You have read my descriptions of what life will look like if you continue on your current path and do nothing about your scoliosis. Now I want to look at the bright side of things. Join me as I describe an alternative to the doom-and-gloom outlook you might be living under.

CHAPTER THIRTEEN

What Does Successful Treatment Look Like to You?

HERE'S AN IDEA: WHAT if you were the person in charge of your scoliosis treatment?

I know that it must seem like you are on a ride controlled by experts who know better than you what is right for your condition. That's not the case, though.

Have you heard of the term *patient-centered* before? It is used to describe medical care that puts the patient first, making them the number one priority of any treatment plan. This should not be such a radical idea, but in our world where patients can feel like numbers inside of massive, uncaring systems, patients rarely feel like they are at the center of their own care.

From my perspective, nothing I do makes sense for my practice if it isn't focused primarily on the patient. My practice at the Scoliosis Reduction Center has many moving parts. It's a business with a bottom line, of course, and it's an employer of a small team of amazing individuals. There's a lot to manage in order for us to be successful at what we do here. But I know that if I move my focus too far away from the people at the center of it all—the patients—the whole enterprise would begin to fall apart.

The reality, for me, is that success is all about the patient. It isn't about my success or the achievements that we accomplish as an organization. It's about individuals like you, people who just want a little bit of hope and some relief from the ever-worsening effects of their scoliosis.

The patient-centered approach to treatment isn't the norm, as I suspect you may have found out the hard way. I can understand if you're feeling frustrated by a system that seems to care very little about the underlying cause of your concerns. This model of health care is so prominent that you may have been unaware that alternatives exist to the reactive type of care you've received in the past. But now you know that it doesn't have to be this way for patients in the health-care system. It can feel as if the traditional medical establishment has betrayed you.

As you know, scoliosis doesn't improve on its own. As a progressive condition, it only places your spine farther and farther out of alignment (and farther from a healthy, normal curvature) over time. Under the traditional model of treatment, doctors watch and wait, taking no action in reducing the curve until the point where surgery becomes the only option on the table. It's kind of a lose-lose situation, isn't it? You can live in pain and severe discomfort until you get the chance to have surgery, which is never guaranteed to work. No one can promise that it will reduce your pain or discomfort. No one can promise that you won't have to undergo additional surgeries. In reality, no one can promise anything at all when it comes to spinal-fusion surgery for your scoliosis.

You should also consider the high risk of complications associated with scoliosis surgery. Although spinal-fusion procedures have become quite commonplace, the rate of complications is rather high. In fact, research indicates that complications may be more prevalent than has been reported previously (*source: https:// www.ncbi.nlm.nih.gov/pmc/articles/PMC2525632/*).

Some short-term side effects and complications of scoliosis surgery include the following:

- excessive blood loss
- nerve damage
- infection
- pain at the site of fusion

Long-term side effects and complications can include the following:

- nerve damage
- back pain
- loss of flexibility
- limited range of motion
- hardware malfunction
- adverse reaction to hardware
- loss of strength in the spine
- strained muscles surrounding the spine
- a spine that's more prone to injury
- emotional stress of living with a fused spine
- financial strain due to surgery cost

Here at the Center, my approach is functional, meaning I prioritize the spine's health and function over curvature size. If I can reduce a patient's curvature through a more natural and less invasive means, the spine's function and health are preserved, whereas a larger curvature reduction achieved through surgery can come at the cost of spinal flexibility, comfort, and quality of life.

Viewed through this lens, traditional treatments actually limit function immediately following surgery or potentially many years down the road. A comprehensive conservative approach works to increase the function of the spine so it can support itself.

Alternatively, you can live in pain and severe discomfort, choose not to have surgery, and then continue to live in increasing pain and discomfort for the rest of your life. And as I mentioned in chapter 10 of the previous section, adults with scoliosis who do nothing to treat the condition have a life span that is as much as fourteen years shorter than the average person.

For you, as the patient, it isn't only helpful to consider what care should look like to you; it's critical to the success of the treatment.

You're an adult, after all. At this stage of life, you are accustomed to having a certain degree of authority over the way your days go and what you do with your time. You're probably no longer in a position where you are taking orders from others or deferring to someone else's expertise. So why would you let a group of strangers decide what's best for you when it comes to treating your scoliosis?

Maybe you assume that it's just the way it has to be. Professionals in the health-care industry have received extensive training, and they've devoted their lives to their respective specialties and occupations. They have advanced knowledge that you couldn't even begin to understand, right?

Well, that's partly true. The amount of knowledge that exists in the brains of today's doctors and other health-care professionals is truly staggering. It's true that the average person couldn't begin to comprehend the vast medical wisdom and terminology that today's professionals carry with them. All of this is true, and yet it doesn't mean that these amazing individuals should be located at the center of your treatment, leaving you on the sidelines.

EVIDENCE BASED CLINICAL PRACTICE

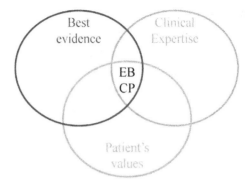

In contrast to the standard model of treatment, my team and I use an approach known as *evidence-based practice*, or EBP. In this three-pronged model, you and your family's values are equally as important as your provider's clinical expertise and the best available evidence for treatment. This approach works because it takes the most important factors into account while considering the best-possible long-term outcomes for you, the patient.

Not all of the knowledge, wisdom, and expertise held by people in the traditional health-care system is up to date, though. Under the traditional model of scoliosis treatment, for example, surgery is still seen as the gold standard of "successful" treatment. Professionals who operate under this model may be aware of alternative treatments, but they don't take them seriously. They've spent countless hours learning, studying, and improving their surgical skills, so it's easy to understand why they wouldn't be advocates of alternatives. Consider it this way: If you were to choose surgery, wouldn't you want a surgeon who has dedicated their career and practice to becoming excellent at surgery? You wouldn't want a surgeon who has also devoted time and energy becoming an expert at conservative treatment options as well.

In my opinion, treatments that don't put the patient at the center can never really be "successful." I've seen a wide range of patients in my practice who have gone through the ringer of the traditional system of treatment. They come to the Scoliosis Reduction Center feeling a little tentative and, to be honest, a little bit wounded by their experiences.

As an adult with scoliosis, it's pretty likely that you know exactly what I'm referring to. In many modern health-care situations, patients like you are treated like numbers, like data points in a completely depersonalized system. If you have sought treatment under the traditional model, you've probably been given very little hope. You have probably never been asked what success looks like to you, either.

I know that on a one-to-one level, your doctors and other providers may be quite encouraging, helpful, and hopeful. They're great at what they do, and it's likely they have inspired confidence in you. Because of this, the depersonalization that so many people feel may not match your personal experience. But your providers, excellent as they may be, still operate under the traditional model, which doesn't always take your concerns and values into consideration.

My Journey to a Patient-Centered Approach

I'm grateful to have traveled down a path that has led me to become a patient-focused provider. However, when I look back, it's easy to see how I might have subscribed to the traditional model of scoliosis treatment if my life had taken some different turns. Luckily, my personality wouldn't allow me to simply go along with the traditional model without questioning it.

I saw countless adults and adolescents diagnosed with scoliosis. They were told that there was nothing that could be done beyond watching and waiting. The most a provider would do under the traditional model was to order periodic X-rays in order to monitor the patient's spinal curvature progression. Of course, medications would be prescribed in order to ease the symptoms of a progressive problem. No action to reduce the curve would be taken. That didn't sit right with me. I can't fault the doctors in these situations; they were highly skilled experts in their fields, doing everything "right," according to the traditional approach.

I got into chiropractic because I was inspired by providers who helped me in my younger years. They treated me as an individual and made me feel like they were personally invested in helping me be my best. I'll never forget the way my life was transformed by caring chiropractic providers.

Given my history, I was completely dissatisfied with the status quo once I learned of the standard watch-and-wait method of treatment. Based on personal experience, I knew that chiropractic care could do amazing things for patients, even those with moderate or severe scoliosis. But I was never going to be able to help those patients if I had remained on the traditional path.

I saw patients being told to watch and wait for years. Inevitably, their abnormal spinal curvatures would progress to the point at which surgery was recommended. Surgery is invasive, expensive, and life-altering. I saw this happening and thought, *We can do better for patients who have scoliosis. Much better.*

These days, my team and I operate under a model that puts the patient first. We believe that the structural condition of the spine must be addressed as soon as possible in order to treat scoliosis effectively. There's no good reason to observe and put off taking action. Rather, once a patient is diagnosed with scoliosis, it's time to begin treatment. Doing anything other than taking action would potentially give the curve more time to worsen. Scoliosis doesn't wait; so, asking a patient to wait while their scoliosis progresses is, in my opinion, completely counterintuitive and counterproductive. It funnels patients toward surgery when surgery should actually be the last resort.

Under the patient-centered model, even those who have severe scoliosis deserve to be treated in a manner that addresses the structural realities of their spines. Waiting longer only ensures that further progression will occur. And although it's definitely possible to work successfully with patients who have severe curvatures, it's always preferable to start treatment before the spine reaches that point.

Treating scoliosis effectively under the chiropractic-centered model requires us to manipulate the spine and move it into a corrected position. Waiting for further progression only makes that process more difficult—for providers *and* for patients.

This chapter began by asking the question "What does successful treatment look like to you?"

Now that you know about functional, patient-centered treatment approaches, I hope that you are challenging yourself to aim a little higher than you have in the past.

Successful treatment of scoliosis in adults will always be based on each individual patient. But I think we can all do better at raising the bar when it comes to the consensus about what can be done with the condition. I believe that the standard treatment model should put patients like you at the forefront. Your voice should be the one that's listened to the most, and treatment goals for your scoliosis should be based on what *you* want, not what surgeons or hospital administrators want.

It isn't necessary to get caught up in a massive, intimidating system as an adult with scoliosis. You don't need to feel like a number or just another data point. You deserve to be in charge of what your treatment plan looks like, in collaboration with your providers.

In many cases, patients picture their futures based on the options their doctors present to them. I think things should be different. In the model I believe in, patients tell their providers what they want their lives to look like. Then the providers craft treatment plans with their patients—specifically for each individual. The collaboration is key; working together with a provider who cares about helping you achieve your ideal future is the best way for you to move forward treating your scoliosis.

In the next chapter, I'll explore these ideas further and explain how you can make sure you're on the same page with the people who can help you achieve the life you want.

CHAPTER FOURTEEN

Getting on the Same Page with the People Who Can Help

A PATIENT-CENTERED APPROACH TO treating scoliosis puts you in the middle of your treatment. For some people, this seems like it might be a lonely proposition. But patient-centered doesn't mean "patient solo." It means that the patient is the hub in a network of people who support them as they treat their condition. It isn't lonely at all, and it ensures that patients like you receive what is necessary to achieve success in their treatment.

When treating adolescents who have scoliosis, it's natural for a team to form around each patient. Parents and other members of the patient's immediate family tend to rally around them, providing emotional support and love. Teachers, counselors, and others from school often step in to lend support too. Adolescent patients can largely focus on their treatment without having to mind the administrative aspects of seeking and receiving treatment; the adults in their lives take on those duties, ensuring that the teenage patient can simply keep their mind on undergoing treatment.

Adolescents represent our hope for the future, so it's easy to see why communities would offer support alongside parents and others close to the patient.

But in cases of adult scoliosis, forming a positive network of helpful individuals isn't always so easy to do.

You have probably experienced this difficulty yourself as you've attempted to rally support around you and your condition. Adults have busy, complicated lives. There are children to raise and jobs to go to every day. And once you reach a certain age, it can seem like all of your peers have some health problem or another, making them less available to provide support by becoming members of your team.

So what can you do to get the support you need as you embark on your journey of treating scoliosis? How can you ask for help? And who are the people you absolutely need in your corner?

Luckily, you probably have family members and friends you know you can trust. These are the people you call when there is big news in your life or when you have something important to share. Don't be afraid to lean on these relationships, even though it may seem like these people have better things to do. The truth is that working through scoliosis treatment is a big deal; the people closest to you should know about the developments that happen as you endeavor to make your life better. Don't just assume that they have too much going on to listen to you or offer understanding.

Also, it's important to remember that the scoliosis treatment journey isn't all hard work, effort, sweat, and tears. There are lots of things to celebrate as you achieve milestones in your treatment. If you cut the people closest to you out of the loop, you lose the chance to share your excitement when you start to see results. If you had a close friend or family member with scoliosis, you would want to be there for them, right? Of course. So don't hide your scoliosis, its treatment or how you feel about the condition. Be open. Advocate for yourself and remember that your journey isn't a solo one, even though you're the person in the middle of everything.

As you connect with the most important people in your life regarding your scoliosis and your plans to treat it, it's also important to keep in mind that people don't always have the most accurate impressions about the condition. As you know, there is a lot of misinformation and misguided opinion about scoliosis. People who know very little about the condition may act like experts or offer "solutions" that you know won't work for you. That's okay. Not everyone needs to be an expert on the condition in order to provide support.

You will likely need to do some education as you go forward through treatment. It may feel like a burden, but it's actually an opportunity to make the world a little bit better for those who live with scoliosis in adulthood. Your story is an important one, just like everyone else's. So it's good to use your voice to explain what the condition is really like for you, and to inform people about concepts like scoliosis-specific chiropractic care, functional treatment, and patient-centered care.

Here's an example: Let's say gardening is your passion. Unfortunately, your scoliosis has progressed to a point where gardening has become more painful than you can tolerate. You've had to reckon with the possibility of a life lived away from your passion and joy. But thanks to scoliosis-specific exercises and your doctor's commitment to a functional-treatment approach, you are able to work toward getting back to the activity you love. Under this approach, you can look forward to the possibility of a reduced curvature and a stronger spine. Under the traditional approach, getting back to the garden might not be possible in a manner that works for you. Stories and examples like this are powerful, and they can broaden people's perspectives on what you're going through.

It can be helpful to talk about scoliosis treatment in terms of what I call *fixed values*. For instance, the surgical approach typically takes only fixed values into account: If there are two patients of the same age with curvatures that are structurally identical, they are likely to receive the same exact surgery. Factors like age and curve structure are fixed values. They and other factors that can be measured, weighed and counted are often the only ones taken into account within the traditional model. This creates a one-size-fits-all method of treatment, which isn't ideal.

My model of treatment takes much more into consideration. *Nonfixed* values such as the patient's occupation, hobbies, activity level, and numerous others are also important. In fact, when taking these factors into account, patients are much more likely to experience a positive outcome from treatment.

If you expect your core friends and family to truly understand the condition the same way you do, you'll probably end up disappointed. You can educate them, and you can be truthful about the way the condition affects you. This will lead to changes in the way your most important people understand adult scoliosis. But remember that the primary role these people should provide is one of emotional support.

Your friends and family can't fix your scoliosis, make your physical pain go away, or prescribe scoliosis-specific exercises. They cannot perform chiropractic adjustments. They can't fit you for a specialized scoliosis brace. But they can provide you with an emotional system of support that allows you to speak freely about what you're going through.

When it comes to the other, more technical, and physically demanding aspects of your treatment, it's necessary to find others to fill in your team's open roster spots.

Building a team around you means finding providers who can help you treat your scoliosis directly. This can be quite difficult because there are so many people who continue to subscribe to the traditional model of treatment for the condition. So although your family and friends don't necessarily need to be experts on scoliosis to help you succeed and provide support, your medical providers should definitely be well versed in the condition and its functional treatment.

How can you locate the right providers and ensure that they'll be positive contributors to your team? Is it possible to tell the difference between providers who specialize in scoliosis and those who don't? I'll explore these topics at length in the next chapter.

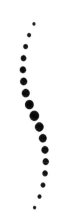

CHAPTER FIFTEEN

Do Your Providers Specialize in Scoliosis?

YOU'RE WELL AWARE OF the challenges of adulthood; I don't need to tell you all about what it's like to be a grown-up in our world—you know all too well what that's about. Not only are you busy with a packed schedule, but also all your peers seem to be in the same position. You also must be your own best advocate. There is no parent or authority figure who will guide you now; it's up to you to make the choices that will serve you best in your future.

And it is up to you to assemble the right team of people who can help you through your treatment of adult scoliosis. Once you have put together your emotional support team, made up of family members and friends, what should happen next?

The first step is finding a specialist who can guide the overall arc of your treatment plan. While you may have been diagnosed by a general practitioner, your primary physician is unlikely to be a scoliosis specialist. Technically, a general medical practitioner can treat you, but they'll be unable to treat your scoliosis, specifically. In reality, any nonspecialist will probably defer to the traditional model of treatment. When it comes to adults with scoliosis, this often means having your symptoms treated without ever addressing the underlying structural issues that are causing them.

Remember: scoliosis is an incredibly complicated condition. Even those of us who understand it on an expert level don't understand it fully. There is much to discover about the nature of scoliosis, how it develops and how it progresses in each individual patient. Because the condition remains relatively mysterious for people who are nonspecialists, seeking out a qualified specialist becomes even more critical to your success.

What we *do* know for sure is that scoliosis is a three-dimensional, progressive condition. It involves all three planes of the spine, which are known as sagittal, coronal, and transverse.

We also know that not all curved spines are caused by scoliosis. Sometimes, things like chronic bad posture can contribute to an abnormal spinal curvature. But bad posture over time wouldn't include the abnormal rotation that would be present in cases of scoliosis. This is just one example of what a specialist might see that a general physician may not.

If you've been diagnosed with scoliosis, that means you have had a Cobb angle measurement of at least ten degrees. Generally speaking, when a patient displays an abnormal Cobb angle, as well as an abnormal rotation, a scoliosis diagnosis is made. This diagnosis may be made by your general practitioner, but again, that doesn't mean they are qualified to treat you and your scoliosis moving forward. In order to ensure that your condition is treated effectively, you must work with providers who, at the very least, acknowledge that your condition is in 3-D. Otherwise, you will find that your scoliosis will continue to progress. Sooner or later, you may be presented with the recommendation of surgery as your next step. And that's exactly what you should try to avoid.

Another undeniable fact about scoliosis is that it's a progressive condition. It doesn't stand still. It doesn't stay static. It progresses. Sometimes quickly. Sometimes slowly and steadily. But it always progresses.

Even though we can all agree that scoliosis is progressive, there is no one who can predict just how a case will progress over time. Certainly, those who aren't specialists in treating scoliosis have no idea what is likely to happen to an individual patient's curvature, other than the fact that it will definitely progress. This is yet another reason why selecting a specialist is so crucial to your ability to treat your condition effectively.

A specialist, preferably one who is trained in a number of different treatment modalities, will be able to treat your condition and not just the symptoms. They will have a more comprehensive understanding of the condition and its nature. They are more up to date on research into the condition as well, and understand the latest methods for treating scoliosis. They can read an X-ray at a level that goes beyond a cursory glimpse, and they're able to craft individual treatment plans.

As you can see, finding a specialist is one of the keys to ensuring that you receive what you need at the center of your treatment. When you can find a specialist you trust, it can feel like a major relief. Yes, locating such a specialist can be a stressful process, but once this person is in place, the rest of your treatment journey becomes far easier to handle.

Before we move forward, I would like to clarify the major difference between treating a patient's scoliosis symptoms and treating scoliosis as the cause.

Understanding this distinction is important because it will ensure that you know the types of questions to ask and the type of specialist to look for who can give you the greatest potential for successful treatment.

If a person with scoliosis were to seek treatment from a general practitioner, they would be receiving general treatment, not scoliosis-specific treatment. What that most often amounts to is a doctor who will treat the patient's symptoms, which are being caused by the curvature. Meanwhile, the curve continues on its course of progression.

This can include pain management with medication or injections, ordering X-rays to measure the curvature's progression and severity, and can also include a recommended exercise regimen for strengthening the back muscles.

These all sound like good things, and on one level, they are. However, they do little to address the structural issue of the curvature, and that's where the treatment approach of a scoliosis specialist will differ.

In my practice at the Scoliosis Reduction Center, I go much deeper than a general practitioner would with our patients. Here, we look at each individual's spine so we can create a custom treatment plan for each patient. Because I am a chiropractor, my treatment involves chiropractic adjustments, which is no surprise. But that's not all a patient receives. Those adjustments are combined with other treatments, including physical therapy, scoliosis-specific exercises, and custom bracing that is designed to push the spine into the corrected position rather than just trying to squeeze the spine. There are a number of ways we treat scoliosis here, but they are all used in service of each individual patient's needs. There are no one-size-fits-all solutions for scoliosis.

Adults with scoliosis are sometimes skeptical of this type of treatment plan. Why? Because, on the surface, it doesn't seem to address the most pressing symptom of all: pain.

Pain management is important. I would never deny that. But treating the symptom of pain without addressing the underlying structural issues causing the pain is a fool's errand. It only leads to more pain down the road as the spine grows further and further out of alignment.

I understand that what you want most of all is to make your scoliosis pain go away. So you might be reluctant to engage in treatment that doesn't relieve your pain quickly. But trust me—we want your pain to go away, too. And my methods of scoliosis treatment have been highly effective at helping patients achieve considerable reductions in their pain levels. They just aren't nearly as easy as taking pain pills.

Scoliosis-Specific versus General Chiropractic—What's the Difference?

It is commonly assumed that a general chiropractor has the qualifications, expertise, and training necessary to address any kind of back problem. General chiropractors are, in fact, qualified to treat a number of issues related to the back effectively, but what about serious, progressive structural conditions like scoliosis?

Ask the average person to define what a chiropractor does, and they are likely to tell you that general chiropractors are "spine doctors." But it's more precise than that. Technically, chiropractors are professional health-care providers who treat nerve issues by making adjustments to the spine. As I'm sure you know, these adjustments can be incredibly helpful to those who suffer from back pain that is caused by conditions such as sciatica, pinched nerves or issues with the spinal disks. Scoliosis, however, is a long-term, chronic condition. Therefore, it requires specialization in order to be treated effectively.

When it comes to issues that affect the average spine, general chiropractors have the tools, techniques, and expertise to treat most conditions effectively. But a spine that is affected by scoliosis doesn't react to normal chiropractic adjustments in a typical fashion. In fact, standard chiropractic adjustments that would be appropriate for a normal spine might not address the needs of a patient with scoliosis. Without specific awareness and training with regard to scoliosis, general chiropractors may simply be unaware of the potential issues they could cause by performing standard adjustments on patients who have the condition. This is one of the main differences between general practitioners and those who specialize in scoliosis.

In reality, traditional chiropractic can be used to provide short-term pain relief for conditions like back pain or headaches, and it can be recommended for such relief in patients who have small Cobb angles and have reached skeletal maturity. However, there is no evidence to support traditional chiropractic's efficacy when it comes to reduction of the Cobb angle. Treating scoliosis requires specific knowledge of the condition and specialized training.

Consider some of the more common chiropractic adjustments. Some of them involve actions like twisting the neck or pushing on the middle of the back, which isn't appropriate for patients who have scoliosis. For instance, let's say your scoliosis has resulted in a loss of your spine's normal backward curve. The common chiropractic technique of pushing on the back to create a more natural curve won't provide long-term relief, even though it may feel helpful at the time of treatment. Patients with scoliosis often experience joint hypermobility in their necks, which reduces stability considerably. For these individuals, any chiropractic adjustments that involve twisting or turning of the neck should be avoided.

This is a tricky topic to discuss because I don't want people to have the impression that all chiropractic care is inappropriate for treating scoliosis. In fact, chiropractic is one of the best modalities available for treating scoliosis as long as it has a scoliosis-specific focus. Regardless of a person's age or the severity of their condition, scoliosis-specific chiropractic can help to reduce the spine's abnormal curvature while improving the patient's ability to live a rich, fulfilling life.

For me, scoliosis-specific chiropractic exists at the heart of my practice. It's a crucial piece of the treatment puzzle, and when it's done alongside scoliosis-specific exercises with physical therapy and specialized bracing, it can keep patients from enduring further progression of their curvatures. It can also keep them from undergoing surgery for their scoliosis, which is always one of my primary goals.

Scoliosis-specific chiropractors like me have the ability to read multiple X-rays and look at other measurements to determine the specific type and severity of a patient's curvature. We take each patient on as an individual, crafting custom treatment plans for them based on their unique characteristics. I cannot stress enough how important it is to treat scoliosis on a case-by-case basis. General chiropractors won't always have this perspective on the condition.

Under scoliosis-specific chiropractic care, adjustments are made with scoliotic spines in mind. For example, I take each patient's physiology into account when preparing to make adjustments. Issues like hypermobility are taken into account, and adjustments are made with great precision to ensure that problem areas are pinpointed without causing harm to more sensitive regions of the spine.

At the end of the day, it's critical to seek a specialist if your goal is to treat your scoliosis using chiropractic care. Scoliosis-specific chiropractors like me understand the condition on a much deeper and more profound level than general practitioners. Again, this is nothing against those who practice general chiropractic—just because they may not be qualified to treat scoliosis specifically doesn't mean they are bad at what they do. Rather, they may be excellent chiropractors who provide real relief for their patients. They just aren't the right people to treat your specific condition.

So, how can you tell the difference between a general chiropractor and one who specializes in scoliosis? In most cases, your provider will make it clear whether they specialize in scoliosis or not. For example, if you visit my practice's website at https://www.scoli-osisreductioncenter.com/, you will see very clearly that we're all about using scoliosis-specific methods to treat our patients.

Anyone who claims to specialize in scoliosis should be able to describe exactly how their methods differ from those of general practitioners. If your provider is unable to answer your questions or describe their expertise with specific regard to scoliosis, it may be time to look elsewhere. With so much on the line, you can't afford to waste time. So it pays to put in the research and ask the right questions.

Remember—you are at the center of your scoliosis treatment. You get to decide who treats you and how they go about doing it. You don't have to take anyone's word for it; you should feel empowered to make those decisions with your best interests in mind. So here's my advice: Take your scoliosis seriously by seeking out treatment as soon as possible. But also make sure that your providers take scoliosis as seriously as you do, and that they have the specific tools, techniques, and training to back it up.

Scoliosis-Specific Certifications

As you search for specialists who take the approach of treating your underlying structural condition versus treating your symptoms, it's important to understand that they aren't all created equal, so to speak.

Some scoliosis specialists have received training in numerous wide-ranging modalities. Others have received training in just one. To me, it's always preferable to trust the expertise of a specialist who draws from multiple areas of knowledge, training, and experience. The best treatment plans approach scoliosis from multiple angles, not just one.

We are able to achieve such great results for our patients here at the Scoliosis Reduction Center because we believe in a varied treatment approach. We don't just use scoliosis-specific chiropractic, nor do we focus solely on physical therapy, bracing, or scoliosis-specific exercise. Because scoliosis is so complex, it is absolutely necessary to approach treatment this way if you want to see success.

I am able to provide these treatments because I have multiple certifications and qualifications.

Back in 2006, I completed my Intensive Care Certification from CLEAR institute, which is one of the world's leading educational and certification centers for scoliosis. I am proud to say that I now sit on the CLEAR Board of Directors, serving as its chairman. Doctors like me who receive certification from CLEAR study natural approaches to scoliosis care extensively. We understand the condition at a level that is much more complex than general practitioners. I recommend looking for the CLEAR certification as you search for scoliosis-specific chiropractors because it indicates that the provider believes in a comprehensive, effective, and evidence-based approach.

I was also one of the first doctors to receive World Masters Certification from the Italian Scientific Spine Institute (ISICO). Additionally, I have the advanced certification in the scientific exercise approach to scoliosis (SEAS) Accreditation Program. Plus, I have a certification from Gomez Orthotic Systems. I am one of the North American trainers for the ScoliBrace system. Furthermore, I am an instructor in Pettibon Systems and am the developer of MaxLiving's *Core Chiropractic* program. I have also added a certification in chiropractic biophysics recently, which has allowed me to continue my education in the field. Additionally, I am certified in certifications come from digital motion X-ray (DMX).

For me, it isn't about stacking up certifications so I can fill my wall with fancy-looking papers. It's about learning as much as I can about scoliosis on a continuous basis so I can provide the absolute highest levels of support and treatment for my patients. There is always more to learn about the condition, and new advancements in understanding and treating scoliosis are being uncovered all the time. Continuing my education while receiving these certifications is all about making sure I can give patients like you the best possible chance at a positive outcome.

As you can see, I have no problem discussing my certifications and what they mean. As you search for your provider, they should be similarly forthcoming about their qualifications. Don't be afraid to ask doctors for their qualifications. Remember: they are there to serve you.

I mentioned some of the certifications I have received. Here is a list that includes those certifications as well as some others you should look for as you search for the right scoliosis-specific provider to treat your condition:

CLEAR—Chiropractic Leadership, Educational Advancement, and Research focuses on advanced methods of diagnosis, rehabilitation, and treatment for scoliosis.

ISICO—The Italian Scientific Spine Institute is an innovative masters certification in the rehabilitative treatment of nonsurgical spinal diseases.

SOSORT—The Society on Scoliosis Orthopedic and Rehabilitation Treatment promotes the advancement of nonsurgical management of idiopathic scoliosis.

SEAS—The Scientific Exercises Approach to Scoliosis is an innovative and evidence-based approach to scoliosis management through physiotherapy scoliosis-specific exercises.

EXPLORING ADULT SCOLIOSIS

ScoliBrace—This is a certification in corrective 3-D bracing.

The Pettibon System—This certification focuses on assessment and rehabilitation practices that rehabilitate the spine and correct problematic posture.

GOSS—The Gomez Orthotic Spine System is a conservative spinal-deformity treatment approach that promotes spinal stability and balance.

CBP—Chiropractic Biophysics is a certification that focuses on spinal rehabilitation and postural correction.

These certifications are all signs that a provider takes scoliosis seriously and understands the importance of specialization for treating the condition effectively. Many doctors don't have any of these certifications. Others have multiples. As you move forward, I would urge you to keep these certifications in mind, and remember that doctors who hold multiple certifications are likely to have much more training and expertise.

One thing I have learned from being a scoliosis-specific provider is that each individual's condition is completely unique. I have not seen two cases of scoliosis that have been alike, nor have I treated any two patients the same way. Every spine is different. Every patient is different. Every single case of scoliosis is different.

Two patients who had very similar cases of the condition in adolescence can have very different cases in adulthood. There are simply too many factors that contribute to the condition, making it impossible to tell how the condition will affect any individual patient.

Because the condition affects each individual differently, finding scoliosis-specific care is paramount if you want to actually achieve improvement and relief. Yes, any doctor can treat a patient who has scoliosis. But not every doctor is qualified to treat the scoliosis itself. That's why general practitioners prescribe pain pills and recommend observation instead of action. More often than not, this type of treatment leads the patient toward surgery as the ultimate attempt to correct the condition. This is just the nature of the traditional treatment model. And I don't think you want that, do you?

If you're reading this book, it's because you know there is more to treating adult scoliosis than what your providers might have been telling you all this time. You're on the right track by seeking out information and learning as much as you can about your condition. Don't you want your providers to have the same approach when it comes to understanding scoliosis?

Scoliosis isn't a network of annoying, irritating, or painful conditions. Yet that is how the establishment tends to treat the condition. Of course, this approach leads to very little improvement in the lives of people who live with scoliosis. You know that the condition is structural and progressive. You know that the symptoms you experience all lead back to your spine. Now it is time to find providers who agree, providers who specialize in scoliosis.

One of the challenges you may run into is the fragmentation of the conservative care system. You may find yourself wondering how to manage treatment that consists of so many different providers and specialists. Patients can become frustrated quickly by having to see an orthopedist, a physical therapist, a massage therapist, an exercise physiologist and an orthotist, all of whom operate in different locations with their own scheduling systems. It's next to impossible to coordinate all of this treatment perfectly, much less ensure that each one of your providers is on the same page with regard to your treatment plan. In fact, treatment providers may be working against each other without even knowing it, making your treatment less successful than it could be.

Maybe you've even done this dance yourself—traveling from appointment to appointment, managing a tight schedule, and hoping each provider understands the goals of your treatment the same way. It's not easy. Or perhaps you've had individual treatments, but they didn't work because they weren't performed in conjunction with other essential aspects of your overall, ideal treatment plan. I see a lot of patients who have become skeptical of the various modes of treatment I use, which is understandable.

To me, the solution is finding a provider who is certified in all the various types of treatment that fall under the umbrella of conservative, functional, patient-centered scoliosis care. This way, your care is managed from a single point, making your life easier and your treatment more likely to succeed.

Finding the right provider can be challenging. And it might seem like a lot less effort to simply surrender to the established model of treatment. Think about your future, though. What do you want out of life? What possibilities do you see for yourself? I don't think you should be afraid to aim as high as you possibly can.

CHAPTER SIXTEEN

A Picture of What's Possible

WE KNOW ALL TOO well what happens when an adult with scoliosis does nothing to treat the condition. In adulthood, scoliosis doesn't just stop its progression just because the body has stopped growing. Instead, it continues to progress in the vast majority of cases. So adults who at one time felt like they could manage their scoliosis almost always reach the conclusion that something must be done about it, especially when pain reaches a point where it prevents the patient from functioning normally.

Experts will recommend things like watching and waiting, and observation, which are really just code words for doing nothing. And we know that doing nothing is the best way to guarantee that your future will be marked by pain, suffering, and the increasing severity of your condition. So even when you do what doctors and other experts tell you to do, you're still doing nothing about your condition.

Treating the condition's symptoms is also not a useful way to move forward if you want to see real improvements in your life. I know that the relief that comes from the absence of pain is powerful, so you may be tempted to use pain pills or other pharmaceutical solutions to address your most concerning issues. But when you consider that the pain is caused by structural issues in your spine, it almost seems silly to address the pain with pills that only go as far as the surface-level symptoms.

We know doing nothing is the standard model of treatment—and we know that it doesn't lead to improved function; it only leads to invasive spinal surgery. So what can you hope for if you take action and treat your scoliosis starting now?

Well, there are no guarantees that functional, patient-centered treatment will work for you. It is possible that scoliosis-specific treatment won't work and your spine's curvature will continue to progress. While this is possible, it isn't likely that scoliosis-specific treatment will have no positive impact on your condition. In fact, scoliosis-specific treatments have been shown to reduce curvatures and restore function, even in adult patients who have severe scoliosis.

One option is to do nothing at all. Another option is to seek out treatment from providers who don't have specialties in scoliosis, which is, in effect, also doing nothing. Under both of these scenarios, your spine is highly likely to continue its progression, causing increasing pain as it does so. So although there are no guarantees with regard to what scoliosis-specific treatment can do for you, why would you do nothing? Especially considering the fact that there is so much evidence to support the efficacy of treatments like scoliosis-specific chiropractic, exercise, physical therapy, and specialized bracing?

I cannot think of a single good reason why an adult with scoliosis should avoid treating their condition. Of course, as a scoliosis-specific chiropractor, I might be a little biased. But my biases come from what I have actually seen and experienced in my decades of experience. They come from what I have seen happen with actual patients. There is a great deal of evidence to support the manner in which I treat patients.

My understanding of scoliosis—and how it ought to be treated—comes from my eagerness to find solutions for patients who couldn't seem to find any relief.

At one time, I was practicing chiropractic with a highly successful practice. There were about fifteen hundred patients coming through my doors every week. I was helping a lot of people, and I had built a reputation as an expert and a well-regarded professional in my field. However, I was having trouble helping patients with scoliosis find relief. I sensed that I could do more than what my training told me was possible, but I didn't know where to begin.

My training, up to that point, taught me that chiropractic could do very little to help patients with scoliosis. At best, my abilities would allow me to help patients manage it as it progressed. I had one patient in particular who was just not feeling any relief, no matter how much I tried to help using standard chiropractic techniques. I was having a difficult time accepting this reality, so I started doing some research.

I discovered that a chiropractic approach to treating scoliosis did, in fact, exist. But it involved much more than just doing standard adjustments. I watched my patient—who had zero success under general chiropractic care—receive alternative treatments over the course of two weeks. I remember being struck by the sheer level of detail in the care my patient received from scoliosis-specific chiropractic care. And I remember how much my patient's life changed as a result of receiving this type of treatment.

I decided that I needed new training and new expertise. I wanted to learn these new approaches to treating scoliosis using chiropractic so I could help patients who wouldn't find effective treatment otherwise. I saw what was possible with my own eyes. I knew that I could provide a new level of relief and hope for my patients with scoliosis.

Today, my practice is centered on an approach that addresses the underlying structural realities of each patient's spine. We don't treat symptoms just to make patients feel better for a short while. Rather, we place patients on a path that leads to continuous healing and relief from their symptoms on a longer-term basis. Simply managing the condition is no longer good enough. These days, my goal is to help patients improve their conditions. I work with them to build strength and regain functionality. In the majority of cases, we are able to reduce abnormal curvatures. And we are able to help patients reduce the amount of pain they experience.

It sounds amazing, and in many cases, it really is remarkable what is possible for patients. But it's important to temper a patient's excitement somewhat in order to manage expectations. So remember these things about what a scoliosis-specific chiropractor can and can't do:

- Can a scoliosis-specific chiropractor heal your scoliosis? No. We can do a lot, and we go far beyond just managing the condition. But we cannot heal scoliosis. The truth is that nothing can truly "heal" the condition.
- Using an approach that is custom-designed for each individual patient can slow and sometimes stop the progression of a patient's abnormal curvature. It's even possible for treatments to reverse the curvature.
- Scoliosis-specific chiropractic treatments are most effective when they're combined with specialized physical therapy techniques, exercise, and corrective bracing in an additive manner.
- Effective treatment takes effort and commitment. Patients should prepare to take part in an intense program where they'll receive a considerable amount of treatment in a brief window of time.

- Once patients receive treatment from a scoliosis-specific provider, they aren't done. In order to maximize the benefits of treatments, patients are directed to participate in at-home treatments, which are directed and designed by their specialists specifically for them.

As you can see, the rate of success for treating scoliosis is higher when a number of different treatments are involved. Does this mean that you have to find a host of different providers, all of whom specialize in scoliosis? Not necessarily. My practice here at the Scoliosis Reduction Center has become so popular largely because we have all the expertise under one roof. Every facet of treatment can be handled by us here, so patients need not travel all over the country (or the globe) to receive the treatments they require.

Specialists like me who have comprehensive knowledge of the condition can also manage your care from afar, helping you to locate and develop relationships with providers who can help carry out your specific treatment plan. You don't have to do it all alone.

Can Adult Scoliosis Negatively Impact Your Pregnancy?

I know that many readers of this book have already experienced the process of giving birth and raising children. But others may be on the other side of starting a family. If this is you, perhaps you have some questions: Is it safe to get pregnant and carry the pregnancy to term? Will the abnormal curvature of your spine cause complications during birth? Should you avoid starting the family you've been dreaming of having your whole life?

The short answer to all these questions is a resounding *no*.

The concerns women have with regard to scoliosis and pregnancy are certainly understandable. Since scoliosis can have such a profound impact on one's internal organs and systems, it wouldn't be surprising if the condition affected a woman's ability to get pregnant or have healthy children. Thankfully, numerous studies have been conducted over the past several decades into this very subject.

Studies have sought to uncover a connection between scoliosis and pregnancy, but there's actually no evidence that the condition can reduce a woman's fertility, lead to an increase in miscarriage, or contribute to other complications during birth. Women with scoliosis in adulthood have normal pregnancies and experience no difference in the manner of giving birth.

Even in cases where patients have large curves, scoliosis has not been shown to have an adverse effect on a woman's ability to become pregnant.

Does this mean that you don't have to inform your obstetrician about your scoliosis? No; they should be made aware of what's going on with your body for a variety of reasons. For one, those who are pregnant and have severe cases of scoliosis should be monitored more closely. They can develop breathing problems and back pain during pregnancy, so they'll require more specialized care.

Additionally, if an epidural is an option, it's important for your obstetrician to know about your scoliosis. That's because it's inserted into your lumbar vertebrae. If the doctor is unaware of your scoliosis, there is the possibility that they won't insert the needle properly.

Ultimately, pregnancy for women who have scoliosis is largely identical to pregnancy in women without the condition. You're safe to start your family, but be sure to inform your doctor that you have scoliosis.

The approach taken by me and other scoliosis specialists is so effective because it goes past the symptoms the patient is experiencing and addresses the condition structurally. Treating the condition this way actually has a goal of improving the function and strength of the spine, which allows patients the ability to get back to living life the way they want. And for adult patients, that can mean living the life they want for the very first time.

According to some of my adult scoliosis patients, this type of treatment changed their lives and gave them a whole new set of possibilities. One patient in her fifties had been experiencing pain in addition to a severely hunched appearance. She had surgery recommended and was prescribed a traditional brace that did nothing to improve her condition; it only made her more uncomfortable. Thankfully, she found me. After undergoing treatment, I'm happy to say that this patient experienced a reduction in pain in addition to a marked improvement in posture and appearance.

Another adult patient of mine was experiencing terribly painful headaches. Seeking relief led to her being diagnosed with scoliosis. This sixty-six-year-old woman had been a big skeptic of chiropractic care her whole life. But she was willing to try anything to relieve the pain she was in from her headaches. Treatment eliminated her headaches and has improved her scoliosis to a measurable degree. According to her, "I didn't realize I felt that bad until I felt so much better."

I could go on with success stories involving adults like you who have scoliosis. There are numerous cases like these, in which patients who didn't expect much ended up getting a great deal of relief from their treatments. So much good is possible with scoliosis-specific chiropractic treatment. What can you expect?

First of all, you should know that you are a completely unique individual (if you didn't know that already). This means that your spine and your scoliosis are nothing like anyone else's. Therefore, the possibilities of what can happen through treatment will always be somewhat unknown.

However, there are some things I am more than comfortable saying about what you can expect from scoliosis-specific treatment in a general sense.

Although specialists like me cannot "heal" or "cure" the condition of scoliosis in adults, patients who have received treatments from scoliosis specialists—scoliosis-specific chiropractors, in particular—have achieved some amazing results.

What specialists like me do is work to prevent the condition from worsening. As an adult with scoliosis, it is critical that you understand that you will always live with the condition. What you should focus on is *how* you go about living with the condition. I have never cured a patient of scoliosis; in fact, no one ever has. But I can tell you I have seen patients go from being completely exhausted and in excruciating pain to living full, active lives. The restrictions that were formerly placed on their lives have been lifted thanks to their commitment to scoliosis-specific treatment.

You should also expect to take time treating your scoliosis. If you're like most adults who have the condition, it has been with you for a long time, even if you haven't felt its effects until recently. In order to experience relief and reduce your spinal curvature, you must commit to the long road; there are no easy, quick fixes when it comes to scoliosis.

To me, successful treatment for a patient who has adult scoliosis could mean a number of things. A reduction in pain. A restoration of functionality. A stabilized curvature. These are just a few markers that indicate possible success. There are many more.

Just remember there's a lot that is possible if you take proactive steps to treat your scoliosis on a functional basis. You can achieve a lot by taking this type of treatment path for yourself. No improvement is guaranteed. But at worst, you would be taking proactive steps to improve your body while avoiding surgery. That's a big win in my book. At best? You could be living a whole new life. The life you've always dreamed of.

You have to take action starting now, though. And you may have to struggle through the temptation to avoid all the difficult work involved in scoliosis-specific chiropractic treatment. Surgery can be very appealing when you are so eager to get rid of your pain.

So, should you have scoliosis surgery after all? The next section delves into this topic in much more detail.

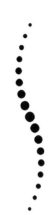

Should You Have Scoliosis Surgery?

USUALLY, ADULT SCOLIOSIS PATIENTS are given only two possible paths to take: One involves the standard, traditional surgery-focused model of treatment. This one will have you watching, waiting, observing and not taking any action. Eventually, this particular path will take you to its final destination—the operating table, where you will undergo expensive and invasive spinal-fusion surgery. This is the path that is overwhelmingly recommended by the established medical model. It's the path that, if you did nothing to advocate for yourself and explore alternatives, you would be placed on automatically. It is the path that the majority of adults with scoliosis are placed on, regardless of the severity of their symptoms or the amount of pain they may be experiencing.

The second path isn't as clearly marked, but it's becoming increasingly well traveled as time goes on. It is the treatment path of the future for adults who have scoliosis. But it's already available today. This less-traditional approach to treatment steers patients away from the possibility of surgery as quickly as possible. Patients like you must take an active role in navigating down this particular road of treatment, but they are guided by scoliosis-focused doctors like me.

I understand why the first path is so popular. Take a look around you, and you will see that, in our culture, we value quick fixes, Band-Aids, and magic pills over treating conditions at their root. Doing nothing allows patients and their doctors to avoid the hard work of actually stabilizing and reducing a patient's abnormal spinal curvature. Ultimately, it may lead patients to surgery, which has its own potential risk of leading to further complications.

In this section, I'll explore the realities of the surgical path—what you can expect, the costs involved, the possible side effects, and more. If you're still considering surgery as a viable treatment option for your condition, I urge you to read through this section thoroughly; you may be presented with some facts that will change your mind.

CHAPTER SEVENTEEN

What Is It Like to Have Spinal-Fusion Surgery for Scoliosis?

LET'S SAY YOU OPT to walk the path of traditional treatment for scoliosis. If you are viewing surgery as the pot of gold that exists at the end of your treatment rainbow, I would advise you to look a little closer at the realities of what a surgical "solution" for your scoliosis would entail. It takes a long time to recover from surgery, for one thing. In fact, many patients don't feel like they have recovered from their surgery until six to twelve months have passed. There are numerous factors that contribute to the amount of time it takes to recover from surgery. Some of those factors extend all the way back to the period of time leading up to your surgical procedure.

What you should be focused on if you travel the traditional treatment path isn't necessarily the surgery you will undergo, but the *healing* from the surgery. Surgery causes a significant amount of trauma to the body, so although it is itself meant to heal a condition, patients often underestimate the amount of healing that has to be done simply as a result of undergoing the procedure. Older

145

patients, for instance, tend to face more challenges in recovery than those of younger age, particularly if they go into surgery with preexisting health conditions.

Here are some of the factors you should pay attention to if you want to maximize your body's ability to heal from spinal-fusion surgery:

- **Mood**—What is your emotional state? If you're an adult with scoliosis, it could be in a delicate condition. It's likely that you've been living in a great deal of physical pain for some time. You have also probably not received the understanding and support you feel you require. For many adults in your position, this can lead to depression or other adverse mental health conditions. Going into surgery with a diminished mood and negative emotional state is never a good idea. Recovering from surgery requires you to be at your best, mentally and emotionally. You will need to keep your mind sharp and positive in order to follow instructions for postsurgical care properly. And you will need to be fully committed to the success of your recovery, which is something conditions like depression can inhibit.
- **Unhealthy Habits**—What has your diet been like recently? Are you getting the proper nutrition, or are you getting by on convenient, highly processed foods? Also, are you smoking or using tobacco? Your level of nutrition is tied directly to your body's ability to heal, so if you aren't eating nutritious whole foods on a regular basis going into surgery, its outcome may not be ideal. Smoking and other forms of nicotine ingestion are also more dangerous than you might expect. Nicotine actually has been shown to inhibit bone growth, which is a necessary process the body

must undergo after spinal-fusion surgery. If you haven't quit tobacco or you're still consuming an unhealthy diet, the chances of surgical success are much lower for you.

- **Obesity**—Diet and smoking can contribute to obesity. Also, a lack of regular exercise is a major contributor. Obesity puts a great deal of stress and strain on the body, which not only contributes to scoliosis symptoms, but also puts patients at greater risk for suffering complications from surgery, whether it is during the procedure or during the recovery period.

As you can see, the state of your mind and body going into surgery is incredibly important. Unfortunately, many adults simply don't have the time, energy, or motivation to tend to these factors appropriately as they prepare for surgery.

Planning and preparing for your surgery involves major factors like the state of your mind and body. It also involves a number of little things that you might not be able to remember so easily.

Preparing for surgery should entail your needs after surgery too. This means making sure your home is set up properly. Do you have a comfortable, easily accessible place to rest? Will you be able to get up and use the bathroom easily? Will you have enough food on hand to feed you? Is the food easy to prepare? Have you arranged for people to check on you or help out around the house as you recover?

Consider the everyday activities and tasks you participate in. Will you need to alter any of those or discontinue them temporarily? Are any of them absolutely necessary? If so, do you have others who can help you with them?

Some of the preparations you make to your home might include installing a toilet-seat riser or handles in the bathroom to make things easier and less likely to cause accidents. You should also make sure you come home to a clean, hygienic house. This will help you avoid the possibility of infection.

Basically, you should take some time to consider what life in recovery will look like. Then, you should organize your home to ensure that it's conducive to your recovery. You will be glad you did, even though there are probably a number of considerations you will miss, no matter how diligent you are.

What Are the Financial Costs of Scoliosis Surgery?

I often refer to spinal-fusion surgery as invasive and expensive. The invasive part is obvious: surgery involves the literal cutting into your body. It is literally an invasion, and your body will treat it as such in many ways; you will experience pain, swelling, and a period of recovery that can last more than a year.

But what about the expensive aspect of spinal-fusion surgery? What are the actual costs involved?

Determining the average cost of a spinal surgery for scoliosis is difficult because there are so many variables involved. Surgeons have experience and they plan for these variables to the best of their ability. Variables can include the location of surgery, the presence of complications and the level of recovery that is necessary. Even the most talented surgeons cannot guarantee the absence of complications during your surgery, and there is a lot that can never be known. So the cost of surgery will vary.

Additionally, the fact that each patient has their own unique version of the condition complicates matters further. But we can come up with some numbers that will help you form your perspective around what you are likely to pay.

The average cost of surgery for scoliosis is anywhere from $140,000 to $175,000, with specific costs breaking down like this:

- 29 percent covers the cost of physical hardware used during the surgery (i.e., wires, rods and screws)

- 20 percent covers the cost of the ICU or in-patient room

- 12 percent goes to the cost of the operating and recovery room

- 8 percent goes to the cost of medical instruments used in the operating room

- 6 percent covers the cost of bone grafting

(Source: http://www.isass.org/pdf/sas11/posters/216.pdf)

Another recent study (https://pubmed.ncbi.nlm.nih.gov/28435918/) that focused on adolescent patients revealed that hospital stays for surgeries decreased by an average of one day from 1997 to 2012. This is a good thing, right? Well, consider that the same study found that the average cost of surgery rose from about $55,000 all the way up to $175,000 over the same period of time. The rate of inflation over that range should have raised the cost from $55,000 to about $79,000. Somehow, an additional $90,000 to nearly $100,000 began showing up on patients' bills to cover the cost of surgery. Patients are staying in hospitals for shorter periods of time, which would indicate that procedures have become more efficient. Yet, they are paying more than twice what they would have paid two decades ago. It just doesn't make sense.

This study didn't take adult surgical cases into account. It's important to note that, in elderly and adult cases, there are more factors to consider, making surgery and other treatments more complicated.

A higher bill for surgery can also come from the presence of comorbidity burden. In other words, when patients had other health problems, it increased the cost of surgery by about $11,000. If these patients required longer hospital stays, it cost them $5,300 more per day. Another factor to consider is the number of levels of spinal fusion necessary. For example, patients requiring more than seven levels experienced an average increase in cost of $65,000.

The bottom line is this: Scoliosis surgery is expensive. Even if your surgery is performed perfectly, you brought no preexisting conditions to the table and your recovery goes according to plan, you're likely to pay well over $100,000. If you are in pain, this might seem like it's worth it. In my opinion, the cost of health care is always worth it if the care corrects problems and provides the desired outcomes. However, surgery is almost always likely to create other problems that will have to be addressed

There are much better options available to you. It is possible to address your condition with functional, nonsurgical treatment that costs much less and offers the possibility of experiencing a much better outcome.

Recovering from Scoliosis Surgery

In the initial couple of weeks after your surgery, you should be receiving the assistance of a friend or family member to help you with the necessities of daily living. This person should be free to care for you without other pressing obligations. If this person can also serve as your transportation provider, that's a bonus. But you should try to limit leaving the house for car rides as much as possible.

You will probably feel exhausted and not quite yourself. In all likelihood, you'll be prescribed pain medications that may leave you feeling drowsy and weak. You need to focus on rest so your body can do what is necessary to recover from the trauma of surgery.

It's important to be extra mindful during this time, even though your mind may be impaired by medications. This is why having a helper present can be so critical to your recovery. For example, there are a number of movements that you should avoid during the initial stages of your recovery. These include bending your back or lifting any object that weighs more than eight pounds. You will benefit by remembering to bend at your knees and hips if you absolutely must reach something. Movements that involve twisting of the spine should be avoided as well. It is especially important to keep this in mind in the morning when you're about to get out of bed. Your natural tendency will be to twist yourself upward to a sitting position, but this should be avoided.

Spinal-fusion surgery involves cutting through your body at a specific incision site. Extra care should be taken with this spot, as it can be conducive to infection. Whenever you take a shower or bathe, you should take time to cover the site of incision carefully. Additionally, you should avoid using any lotions, creams, or powders around the incision site, as they can cause irritation.

After a couple of weeks have passed, life will become a little less restrictive for you. At this time, your incision site should be healed past the point at which infection is possible, which means you can expose it to water again and resume normal bathing. The strength of your pain medication will probably be reduced around this time as well, giving you a little more clarity and energy. This can feel like turning the corner for patients who have been in a medicated fog in the weeks after surgery. You may feel energized and empowered to start living your normal life again, but it's important to take things easy and limit your activity.

At about the six-week mark, you will have X-rays taken of your spine in order to check on the fusion's progress. Your energy levels will continue to rise, but you won't be back to normal yet, in terms of your stamina. Your doctor may lift some additional restrictions at this time. In many cases, this means clearing the patient to drive again. However, your surgeon may recommend a course of physical therapy prior to lifting such restrictions. They will want to observe factors like your reaction times, pain levels, and coordination before giving you the green light to get back behind the wheel or engage in other activities that engage the whole body.

Remember: this is just an average path of recovery. You may be able to resume many "normal" activities after about six weeks postsurgery. But you may require additional time to recover before your doctor is willing to lift restrictions. Everyone is different, and every individual has a different recovery experience after undergoing spinal-fusion surgery.

In about six months to a year after your surgery, you will receive X-rays to determine how well the fusion has taken hold. In many cases, patients' spines are considered fully healed from the surgery. At this time, doctors will allow most patients to return to their normal lives and regular daily activities.

There is a chance that life will never be quite the same as it was before surgery, though. Some activities may never be safe to resume, or they'll require modifications in order for you to participate in them safely. In any event, the nature of the spinal-fusion surgery means that your back won't be able to bend the same way it did before. This means you should be cautious when attempting to return to physical activities that you engaged in prior to surgery.

You should also keep in mind that now is a good time to examine some of your old habits. If you were a smoker prior to surgery, should you go back to cigarettes once you have recovered? Absolutely not. Just because you've experienced "successful" surgery for your scoliosis doesn't mean that you have a pass to ignore your health for the rest of your life. In fact, the opposite is true—if you've had a spinal-fusion surgery for scoliosis, maintaining good health for the rest of your life should be a top priority. Otherwise, you could require additional surgeries, develop physical or mental complications and experience a significantly reduced life span.

After reading all of this, does surgery still seem like a valid option? Does it seem preferable to functional treatment? Does it create a new normal that you can live with? I have a feeling the answer to all these questions is a resounding no.

CHAPTER EIGHTEEN

Surgery Creates a New Normal; What Will that Mean for You?

WHEN ADULTS WHO HAVE scoliosis opt for a surgical solution to their condition, they tend to do so while looking forward to visions of normal life. But is it really possible to have a normal life after spinal-fusion surgery? Can a patient who once lived a vibrant, healthy life return to their former existence? It's not that simple. The fact is that undergoing a major surgery creates a new version of normalcy in the lives of patients.

Keep in mind that adult scoliosis surgery is typically not recommended by surgeons—it is offered as a last resort treatment that comes with a host of complications. Surgeons are reluctant to operate on adult patients because the chances of success aren't particularly high. As a patient ages, the potential rate of complications rises as well, making surgery even less of a viable option. With this in mind, it may be difficult to imagine a new normal that looks like a healthy, vibrant, and active life.

I won't tell you whether your new normal is worth pursuing or not. I just want you to know the facts. I know that the promise of relief from surgery can be incredibly powerful, so much so that patients ignore the possibilities of what might happen if things don't go exactly according to plan. You may feel like undergoing expensive, invasive scoliosis surgery is worth it—thousands of people make the same assessment every year, so you're far from being alone in your decision. The pain associated with scoliosis as an adult can be absolutely excruciating, so I understand the choice to look at surgery as a savior. It's just important that your vision of what surgery entails matches reality.

Surgery can lead to a number of hardships that come as surprises for patients, especially those who thought the surgical path would be easier and less demanding than the functional-treatment model. Many patients explore the functional model through research, but determine that the amount of participation and work that's required of them is just too much to handle. But the difficulties associated with a functional approach to treatment pale in comparison to what is possible when surgery is selected.

Patients who opt for spinal-fusion surgery see the procedure as an operation, which assumes that it's a one-time event. But I would urge patients to view the procedure less as an operation, and more as an *installation*. This brings a whole new set of implications. For people who have scoliosis, spinal-fusion surgery involves the installation of hardware to ensure that the vertebrae hold together as they fuse into a straightened alignment. It's a complex process that often leads to the necessity of more surgeries down the road.

The reality is that outcomes don't always match the visions of success that patients have in their minds. Second surgeries to remove or alter hardware are often recommended after fusion has taken place. And with more surgery comes the risk of greater complications. Furthermore, surgery for scoliosis ultimately leaves the condition untreated from a structural standpoint. This means that many spinal-fusion surgeries are no more than cosmetic procedures. Yes, surgery can stabilize the spine, but what does it really mean for it to be stabilized when surgery can result in chronic pain, disability, and disfigurement?

The truth is that spinal-fusion surgery for scoliosis does little more than transform a patient's spinal deformity into a state of permanent spinal dysfunction. This is the new normal.

Here are some additional facts about what normal looks like for people who have undergone spinal-fusion surgery for scoliosis:

In a study that examined X-rays of patients who underwent surgery twenty-two years prior, it was found that many spines returned to levels of curvature that were present before surgery (https:// pubmed.ncbi.nlm.nih.gov/11242379/)

Each year, roughly eight thousand individuals who underwent scoliosis surgery in their adolescence are designated as permanently disabled. (https://pubmed.ncbi.nlm.nih.gov/12226771/)

Although patients often enter surgery with the expectation that their spines will become perfectly straight and regain full function, the best surgery is expected to do is provide a 66 percent reduction in curvature. The return of full function is never expected by doctors or experts, regardless of the success of the surgery. (https://pubmed.ncbi.nlm.nih.gov/12226771/)

Surgery is also often accompanied by many potential side effects, which can include the following:

- intestinal obstructions
- pancreatitis
- gallstones
- impairment of lung function

- dislodging of hardware hooks
- breakage of hardware rods

Furthermore, patients can become increasingly restricted in their activities after surgery. This is because a spine that is "corrected" and placed in alignment through hardware (rather than through structural correction) is less able to distribute impact and force in an even manner.

There is also the issue of fear and anxiety, which many patients are surprised by after surgery. They worry about their spines snapping or their internal hardware malfunctioning. They find themselves unable to trust their bodies, postsurgery, which limits their ability to participate in activities they love. This creates a cycle that keeps patients inactive, at home, and living in fear. And that's exactly what they hoped to avoid by undergoing surgery for scoliosis.

Why am I discussing the realities of surgery in such detail? Shouldn't I be promoting the effectiveness of functional treatment rather than knocking surgeons? Well, for as long as functional treatment is considered an alternative to the surgical standard, I believe it's important to inform patients about the realities they may face by going under the knife to treat their scoliosis. In the world of medicine, as treatments increase in invasiveness, they are less likely to be performed. Alternatives are sought to the invasive treatment instead. However, in the scoliosis world, this approach seems to have flipped: surgery should be seen as the alternative when functional approaches fail, not the other way around.

My intention isn't to criticize the professionals who have devoted their lives to becoming spinal surgeons. Rather, it is to ensure that people like you have all the information available before making a decision.

Surgery for scoliosis will always be an option, no matter how much I discuss the negative impacts it has. There are readers of this book who may opt, ultimately, to undergo surgery. I just want to make sure they know what they can expect.

Some Notes on Lung Function, Life Expectancy, and Scoliosis

Your thoracic spine is a component of your rib cage, which contains and protects vital organs such as your heart and lungs. That is why scoliosis can sometimes affect the function of these organs. For individuals with scoliosis curves greater than seventy degrees, it can cause difficulties that impact daily life negatively.

According to a fifty-year study (https://pubmed.ncbi.nlm.nih. gov/12578488/), 22 percent of patients complained of shortness of breath, compared to 15 percent of individuals in the control group. Severity of the condition has also been found to contribute to an increased risk of shortness of breath.

In another study, it was found that lung and heart function was correlated significantly with the severity of the patient's scoliosis (hhttps://www.ncbi.nlm.nih.gov/pmc/articles/PMC4510355/).

An additional study (https://www.ncbi.nlm.nih.gov/pmc/articles/ PMC463231/) examined twenty-four scoliosis patients—none of whom had surgery for their condition—in both 1968 and twenty years later. Researchers wanted to know if any changes in lung function had occurred in the intervening years. They found that the changes in lung function that occurred were consistent with those that would naturally occur over that time period as a result of aging. The strongest predictor of developing respiratory failure later on was the patient's lung-function measurement taken back in 1968. The next-strongest predictor was the size of their curvature. Researchers found that only the patients who had low lung function (below 45 percent) in 1968 and also had curves greater than 110 degrees developed respiratory failure later in life. This allowed them to conclude that respiratory failure develops in adults with large scoliosis curves and low lung function who also experience the normal effects of aging on their respiratory systems.

Scoliosis surgery might be attractive to those who worry about developing such respiratory issues in the future, but does it actually work? No. There is little to no improvement that can be expected by undergoing spinal-fusion surgery for scoliosis.

Why am I singling out the lungs? Physicians contributing to the massive, long-term Framingham heart study (https://www.ncbi.nlm.nih.gov/pmc/articles/PMC463231/) have concluded that the condition of a patient's lungs are the top contributor to that person's death. There is a significant correlation, as it turns out, between lung health and one's ability to live a long, healthy life.

In other words, the health of your lungs is a great indicator of what your life span will be. If you have a large lung capacity, you are more likely to live a longer life.

Scoliosis affects your lungs and their function, so it makes sense to treat the condition in order to reduce the strain on internal organs. However, surgery isn't an effective treatment at all when it comes to improving lung function. If your lung function is bad now, it's highly unlikely to improve via surgery. That is another reason why functional-treatment methods are preferable to the standard approach that involves surgery.

Your new normal after surgery will extend into the rest of your life, which may not be a fact you're considering while contemplating surgery. Unfortunately, predicting what your life will look like is difficult to do with any accuracy. Some patients may perform quite well for quite some time after surgery. They feel their lives have improved. Many of them describe surgery as the best decision they made for themselves and their bodies. These descriptions often come from what I call the "honeymoon stage" following surgery. For adolescents, this phase can last a long time, reinforcing the belief in the surgery's effectiveness. But in cases of adult scoliosis surgery, this phase can be all too brief. These surgeries involve hardware, which always has a life span and will more than likely require revision in the future. In other words, additional surgeries could be recommended.

Some patients don't even get to experience the postsurgery honeymoon stage. They complain of mobility issues, trouble sleeping, and increasing amounts of pain. The truth is that it is impossible to tell on a long-term basis how surgery will affect you. It's highly variable.

I have a unique perspective as a proponent of the functional, nonsurgical approach to scoliosis treatment. I'm in a position to see exactly what happens after scoliosis surgery. Why? When patients who have had surgery start experiencing side effects, pain, and other problems, they often reach out to me for help.

In addition to examining numerous patients who have had problems postsurgery, I have collaborated with a wide range of doctors, surgeons and other experts over the years. Taking all of the information into account, a consensus has been reached with regard to the life span of a "successful" scoliosis surgery. That life span is just twenty to thirty years for adolescents, and much shorter for adults (increasingly so as they age). That is a period of time long enough to ensure that patients will have issues, one way or another, related to their surgery. It's just a matter of when and how severe those issues will be.

Invasive surgeries, such as spinal-fusion surgery, that involve the installation of hardware into the body almost always lead to issues down the road. If you have ever had a knee or shoulder surgery, you probably know what I mean. The relief that is felt is typically offset by complications and issues that wouldn't have arisen without surgery.

From what I have observed, the complications that arise from surgery tend to be understated by surgeons and others involved in the traditional orthopedic model of scoliosis treatment. Your surgeon may mention the possibility of side effects or complications, but it is unlikely that they will delve deeply into those subjects with you. In reality, no one can really be sure what is likely to happen after surgery. Long-term effects vary considerably, and the way surgery impacts each individual patient is different. What's more, the life span of the rods and other hardware used in surgery cannot be predicted accurately.

You might be expecting your new normal after surgery to include some cosmetic improvements, too. Like many patients who opt for spinal-fusion surgery, you may be assuming that your body will become more symmetrical, allowing you to expand your wardrobe and show off your figure. But you're likely to be disappointed by the results you achieve. In reality, the goal of scoliosis surgery is to stop the progression of your spine's abnormal curvature; reducing the curve isn't usually a primary objective. That means you should probably temper your expectations with regard to any possible cosmetic improvements following surgery.

Surgery might give you an improved physical appearance, but in all likelihood, you will appear more or less the same as you did before surgery. If you think your waist asymmetry or rib deformity will go away after surgery, you may be in for an unpleasant surprise.

As an adult with scoliosis, you're probably more concerned with pain relief than any possible improvements to your appearance. But if there is any part of you that is looking forward to a new, more attractive body shape in addition to your pain relief, there may be some disappointment in store for you. Surgery is very serious business, so you should not put yourself at risk for any amount of potential physical improvements.

Psychologically speaking, you may have some high expectations for surgery as well. Even if your surgery is completely successful, you'll go through some emotional, psychological ups and downs that may be difficult to deal with. Such an invasive procedure not only takes energy from your body, but also takes a toll on your psyche. And the fact that spinal-fusion surgery leaves a metal rod in your body is one that your mind will wrestle with long after you've undergone the procedure.

Surgery comes with lifelong psychological consequences that you must be prepared to deal with. Sweeping your emotions under the rug is a sure way to make them come back stronger and more difficult to cope with. So you should not go into surgery thinking that life will ever be the same as it was before the procedure.

Your life will involve a tremendous amount of monitoring and observation after surgery. If you thought all the watching and waiting before surgery was bad, I'm sorry to say that you'll have to endure a lot more of it once you've had surgery. Doctors need to make sure that you're free from infection and that the hardware installed in your body is operating properly. They'll also monitor the degree of your curvature to make sure it isn't progressing. Although you may not expect your spine's curvature to progress at this time, it isn't uncommon to still notice changes in curve size after surgery.

As far as limitations on your life are concerned, you always have to be on alert. Your body is different after surgery than it was before it. You're likely to be a bit more fragile and delicate. Injuries may occur more frequently under stress and strain. Recovery from those injuries might take a little longer and be a little more difficult to endure.

There may also be a small part of you that worries about the state of your spine. Hardware failure is a real thing—rods can break or screws can loosen—and you may always be tentative when it comes to participation in physical activities. This low-level hum of worry may not amount to much, but it will always be there in the background, affecting the way you go about your life.

Think about the latter stages of your life and how you want it to look. It's possible to live your entire life with scoliosis and develop quite a large curve without experiencing any limitations to your life. I have seen many such patients here in my practice. They have endured pain and suffering, to be sure, but their lives are almost certainly better off than if they had undergone surgery, at least in terms of the limitations they live with.

The fact is that surgery is a point of no return. There is no going back to a life before spinal fusion. And there are no guarantees that, once you've had a surgery, you will need no more.

There are also effective alternatives to surgery. So the choice isn't to act or not act; rather, it should be a choice regarding the specific action you want to take to address your condition and improve your life.

Functional Treatment Postsurgery

Earlier in this chapter, I mentioned that I have seen patients who have reached out to me after experiencing issues related to their spinal-fusion surgeries. They experience complications and side effects that, for whatever reason, have not been addressed by providers under the traditional model of treatment. They are frustrated and often angry. They want answers and they want real relief.

I am happy to help these individuals, and I'm glad that their paths have led them to me and my practice. But I always wonder about these patients and where they would be had they avoided surgery and received functional, patient-centered treatment instead.

Again, surgery is permanent, so there many of the improvements that would have been possible prior to surgery are just not available after the fact. That being said, there are options for these patients. It's important to manage expectations, though. Predicting outcomes from treatment is nearly impossible. There is a lot of uncertainty to deal with, largely because there's so much potential variance in the nature of the surgery itself.

Each surgeon has their own individual preferences and ways of doing things. Surgeons don't all subscribe to the same techniques, nor do they all use the same sets of standard tools. Hardware preferences differ, and even the length of the rods is subject to a particular surgeon's preferences.

There is also the factor of *when* a person had surgery. Even though very little has changed with regard to spinal-fusion surgery as a treatment for scoliosis, there have been a few advancements made over the years. New techniques have appeared, and new hardware innovations have arrived on the scene. For example, the invention of the pedicle screw has reduced surgical hardware failures considerably. When a patient experiences complications, it's necessary to take all the potential variables into account in order to provide a prognosis.

Essentially, it is very difficult to predict the results of chiropractic-focused treatment for those who have had prior spinal-fusion surgery. We must modify the approach we take with these patients, which limits their maximum effectiveness. It's also of paramount importance to help patients avoid additional complications or surgeries, so our treatments aren't as aggressive as they would be for those who have not had surgery.

I have to admit, though, that even given the difficulties of treating individuals who have had spinal-fusion surgery, it is worth it. It's possible for us to help these patients find real relief and begin to live their lives fully again. I just wish they had found me sooner, before deciding to undergo surgery.

The new normal of life after scoliosis surgery is different for everyone. And it is usually far different from the old normal for each patient. There is also not enough data available to say, for sure, what the long-term effects of surgery are.

There have been studies showing what happens after surgery, but in most cases, those studies only extend five years past the date of the operation. For adults, there's even less available data. They aren't reliable, so it's difficult to glean any concrete information from them. There really is a considerable gray area when it comes to what we know about life after spinal-fusion surgery.

Though there is still a lot to uncover about life after spinal-fusion surgery, we do know some things for sure. One of them is surgery is invasive and always carries with it risks and the possibility of complications. It's also true that the results of surgery are often lost not long after surgery, and if you're an adult, you run a much greater risk of experiencing complications.

I know that you probably just want to make your pain go away right now. You want a fix for your condition, preferably one that doesn't involve a ton of effort on your end. I get it. But I think it's important to consider your life beyond surgery. You may continue to experience pain and suffering. You're likely to suffer some kind of side effect or complication. You will introduce limits to your life that may never be removed. Is it worth it?

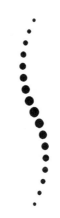

CHAPTER NINETEEN

Surgery Isn't the End of Your Scoliosis Story

IF SURGERY IS YOUR end goal for treating scoliosis after years of painful watching and waiting, I'm afraid I have some bad news for you: Surgery is just the beginning of a new story for you.

Metal rods are inserted into your body during spinal-fusion surgery. These pieces of hardware are engineered to act like splints that hold your spine in a corrected position during the actual fusion process. It takes about six months for this to happen, but the fusion itself could be occurring for a full year. Your bones, having been fused together in this process, attempt to prevent your spine from curving abnormally. Those metal rods remain inside your body, though, because you would need to have another surgery to take them out.

The whole process of recovery takes time; usually more time than the patient is prepared to take. Returning to a "normal" life doesn't happen overnight. It might not happen at all.

Limitations, pain management, and the need to have assistance from others are all common factors for those who are in the recovery period from spinal-fusion surgery. Usually, patients are prescribed medications that take the pain away, but they also reduce cognitive ability and energy levels. It isn't a fun time; it can be even more difficult to deal with than the effects of scoliosis.

There is also the issue of the surgical incision site, which can be vulnerable to infection. It is difficult—if not totally impossible—for patients to dress this site themselves prior to showering or bathing. It's just another reason why having a friend or family member around to help you is so crucial to your recovery.

Follow-up appointments will begin to dot your calendar starting at about two weeks following your surgery. Doctors will examine you to determine how well the fusion is doing. You also have an opportunity at this time to ask questions and let your providers know how you're feeling. You're just starting your recovery at this time, and there's still a long road of recovery in front of you.

Why Is the Surgical Model of Treatment So Dominant?

The traditional medical approach to treating scoliosis has been established for decades. Dislodging the status quo can be highly difficult in the world of medicine, even when alternative treatments have been shown to produce more beneficial outcomes. I am happy to say that functional-treatment options, such as pursuing scoliosis-specific chiropractic, are becoming increasingly popular and well known among patients and the general public. And yet, the dominant treatment approach continues to be regarded as the standard.

I believe there are a number of key reasons for this.

For one, doctors are often reluctant to recommend alternative treatment options to patients. These options will remain unacknowledged by your provider at best. They may be laughed at, at worst, if you happen to suggest them as treatments that could be effective while you watch and wait.

I know that many patients perform research into alternative treatments, just like you are doing now. They present these treatments to their providers only to be told that they are a waste of time. As you know, that isn't even close to the truth.

Providers under the established medical model of treatment aren't necessarily acting nefariously when they discourage you from seeking alternatives. They are just so entrenched in their model and approach that anything else seems absurd to them. To them, watching and waiting (and, eventually, surgery) are completely legitimate treatments for your condition.

Another factor that makes the surgical model so dominant is the decrease in frequency of screenings for scoliosis. The logic behind not screening says there is nothing you can do to prevent curve progression; therefore, it makes no sense to screen for a condition that cannot be improved.

Screening is obviously important in terms of detecting the condition as early as possible. When it comes to treating scoliosis, early detection is always critical to success. So it's a good thing that people get screened to see if they have the condition. Unfortunately, as a result of reduced screening efforts in adolescents, many cases don't get diagnosed until the curve has reached a level requiring surgery.

The average curve size for which surgery is considered necessary has decreased from 60 degrees to 42 degrees. Effectively, this change created situations in which more and more people were considered qualified for surgery. This has led to an increase in the number of surgeries performed, which has, in turn, reinforced the belief that surgery is the gold standard of treatment.

Consider what typically happens when a person receives a scoliosis diagnosis too—the patient is referred to an orthopedic surgeon for management. In this scenario, it is hard to imagine a patient ending up anywhere but in surgery. On the other hand, when a patient's case is managed by a provider who specializes in conservative treatment, surgery is almost never viewed as an option.

Yet another factor influencing the dominance of the surgical model is the sheer number of surgeons that exist today.

Back in 1941, the United States population included one orthopedic surgeon per every 110,000 citizens. In 1999, that number changed to 1 out of every 15,150 citizens. Naturally, the more surgeons there are in the world, the more surgeries that will be performed. It also means that many surgeries are taking place that may not be medically necessary.

Surgery should be a choice made by you after performing research, talking to trusted people and weighing what is best for you and the life you want to live. Sadly, our dominant surgical model of treatment for scoliosis makes that choice quite difficult for people like you.

Your spine's abnormal curvature is unique, and there's no other scoliosis patient who has the condition in the same exact way you do. That being said, there are some scenarios I see play out commonly after scoliosis surgery. Here's one I challenge you to picture yourself living:

Months go by after your surgery. You become increasingly anxious as you hope to get back to some kind of normalcy in your life. However, you need to continue treating your recovery seriously. This is particularly true if you have begun to let normal activities trickle back into your daily life. You may be getting out of the house more, and you will no longer be addled by such strong medications. But you have to stay smart about your recovery so you can ensure the best-possible outcome.

In the months and years that follow, you experience moments when you may feel fully recovered. However, there will also be many moments when you feel the effects of surgery. While you will be able to resume many activities, your body won't allow you to resume others, depending on the way your spine heals from surgery. You could have a completely successful surgery and still experience side effects and long-term issues years down the road.

Of course, no one will be able to tell you with any certainty what life will look like after you have undergone spinal-fusion surgery. Every individual has their own story and their own set of specific circumstances that they bring with them. The way scoliosis manifests in one person could be much different than how it manifests in you or anyone else. You may undergo surgery and experience very few side effects or complications. Or you may undergo surgery and experience every side effect and complication possible. There really is no way to tell.

Even if every aspect of your surgery goes perfectly by the book and your recovery goes extraordinarily well, you could still experience issues years down the road. Many patients initially view surgery as a cure or an endpoint, but it isn't that; it's a new beginning. While your scoliosis symptoms might recede after surgery because your spine has been stabilized, surgery is likely to introduce a number of potential issues, some of which could be even more troubling than dealing with scoliosis.

Is this what you want for yourself? Do you feel comfortable living a life that trades scoliosis symptoms for surgical side effects and complications? Or are you willing to take a different path? A path that puts you in the driver's seat. One that avoids surgery. It is possible.

Not long ago, there were no effective alternatives to the standard, surgery-focused model of scoliosis treatment. But things are changing rapidly. In my role as a scoliosis-specific chiropractor and leader in my field, I have been advocating for the adoption of alternative treatments for quite a while. Thankfully, these types of treatments are becoming more widely recognized. And it's easy to see why functional treatment of scoliosis is so attractive to people—we don't watch and wait for a curve to grow even larger and more difficult to deal with. We get to work right away with our patients, putting in the work that can actually reduce a patient's spinal curvature and allowing them to experience relief without surgery. My methods may not be as well-established as the traditional model, but they are on their way.

CHAPTER TWENTY

Surgery Is No Longer the Gold Standard of Scoliosis Treatment

WHEN THE AUTOMOBILE WAS first introduced, many people were afraid of it. They didn't see how it would be possible for people to travel at speeds greater than 25 miles per hour without putting themselves in great physical danger. The advent of the automobile made peoples' lives easier and more efficient. It was truly revolutionary. And yet, there were people who feared the new invention, believing that the horse and buggy was the gold standard of transportation.

These days, it's impossible to imagine a world without cars. They are the standard model of transportation. Most people wouldn't be able to live their lives the way they do now without cars. They have become absolutely essential. In fact, cars have transformed from objects of mistrust to ordinary, everyday transportation tools.

I wonder if the trajectory of functional, patient-centered, and noninvasive treatment for scoliosis might take a similar path to becoming ordinary. These days, people are highly skeptical of the treatment methods employed by chiropractors like me and other scoliosis-focused providers. They are skeptical even though the evidence to support the efficacy of alternative treatments grows each day. No amount of success stories will convince some people that there are better methods for treating scoliosis than surgery. But more and more people are learning about these methods, trusting them, and living their lives proudly after undergoing functional treatment. The tides are shifting. The standard for treatment of scoliosis is shifting too, slowly but surely.

People in our society have been conditioned to view surgery as a fix for certain medical issues. It's not just scoliosis, either; it is common for people to treat symptoms and engage with their health issues on a surface level without treating underlying conditions. Eventually, these issues become severe to the point where invasive treatments like surgery become "necessary."

The fact is that it's getting harder and harder to convince people that surgery should be the focus of their treatment. People are learning about the value of active living, a healthy diet, and restorative sleep. They are more aware of the connections between their choices and their health than ever before. They are becoming increasingly open to alternatives when it comes to their health care. In my mind, this means that surgery is already far from being the gold standard of scoliosis treatment. It's just taking a while for the powers that be to catch up with what you and I know: surgery is far from the best option for treating scoliosis.

One of the issues with the prevalence of the surgical model is that its dominance makes people think surgery is no big deal, like it's normal to undergo such an invasive procedure. It is the default approach and has been for decades. This model of treatment became so entrenched that people stopped understanding the realities of surgery.

Spinal-fusion surgery for scoliosis is an extremely serious procedure. It should not be taken lightly. It's a life-altering event that cannot be reversed. Although it has become the standard for treatment, I believe it's important for patients like you to know the truth. I want you to know that you have options that don't involve surgery.

Surgery will always be around, and it will always have its place. My concern is that it has become a cure-all for any condition when it should only be a last resort. Alternative approaches used by scoliosis-focused providers like me are effective without being invasive or expensive like surgery.

I have a bias toward alternative treatments that don't involve surgery, and I am fully willing to admit it. But my bias is based on decades of training, experience, certification, and working with patients from all over the globe. It's based on the results I have actually seen in my practice at the Scoliosis Reduction Center. Patients arrive, sometimes feeling scared or confused about their condition. They believe that surgery is their only option, but they don't want that. They are wary of watching and waiting, and they know in their guts that there must be another way.

I give patients the perspective that they don't always have access to elsewhere. Certainly not if they have been receiving treatment from the standard medical model. I also give patients hope; or rather, I help them find the hope that was in the all along. If the treatment methods we use don't work, surgery is always an available option—I think it's important that patients know that. However, it is rare, once a patient has begun their treatment, to ever consider the surgical path seriously unless it becomes medically necessary. It becomes obvious that surgery is far from being the standard it was once thought to be.

Still not convinced that surgery should become an outdated model for treating adult scoliosis?

Here are some facts:

Spinal-Fusion Surgery Cannot Cure Scoliosis

Spinal-fusion surgery can stabilize the spine and provide some relief for patients. But it cannot cure the condition.

Honestly, nothing can cure scoliosis. The condition, once it's present, always remains in the body. There is no procedure or therapeutic method that can eliminate it. There are no medications that can treat it structurally, which is how it must be treated in order to experience any level of effectiveness.

Having surgery for scoliosis doesn't return the body to anything resembling a normal state, even though surgery can sometimes result in what appears to be a reduction in curvature. What if you were experiencing pain in your elbow and had surgery that fused your arm joints completely? Would you consider that a success? Probably not, because your arm would have its function limited severely.

Surgery doesn't address the underlying structural issues at the core of the condition. It actually introduces new issues, side effects and complications, potentially. Successful surgery is also no guarantee that the scoliosis won't continue to progress, making additional surgeries necessary.

Spinal-Fusion Surgery Will Probably Not Improve Your Mobility

In fact, it might reduce your mobility.

Many adults with scoliosis have been conditioned to believe surgery is the thing that will make every aspect of their lives better. They have become so accustomed to thinking of surgery as the ultimate scoliosis solution that they fail to consider some of the troubling side effects involved. In reality, it is unlikely that a patient will be able to return to the same levels of mobility, postsurgery, that they experienced prior to it. Often, patients notice a decrease in their mobility levels.

Studies have shown some concerning results with regard to patients' mobility after surgery. In this study, it was found that mobility actually decreases by an average of about 25 percent after a patient has undergone spinal-fusion surgery. (https://pubmed.ncbi.nlm.nih.gov/16449904/)

Another study showed that the decreases in mobility experienced by patients after surgery didn't go away quickly. In fact, they remained after as much as twenty years elapsed. (https://pubmed.ncbi.nlm.nih.gov/16449899/)

Surgery is permanent. Its effects are permanent. Some of those effects will be desirable, such as the stabilization of the spine. But many of them will haunt you for the rest of your life. So before you decide to undergo surgery for your scoliosis, remember this.

In Spinal-Fusion Surgery, Disks Are Removed from the Spine

Did you realize that when you undergo spinal-fusion surgery, the surgeon actually removes disks? These disks are crucial to your anatomy, but they are technically not essential for the body's ability to function. For some people, the removal of spinal disks means the absence of vital shock-absorbing properties in the body. Subject to strong or traumatic force, the body cannot handle impact in the way it once was able to. Car accidents, for example, can cause shock and trauma that transfer tremendous amounts of force down the surgical rods implanted into the body, potentially causing a great deal of damage.

This is the reality of surgery. It's permanent. It changes people. And it doesn't always improve a patient's life.

How Did We Get Here? A History of Scoliosis Surgery

How is it that surgery became the gold standard for scoliosis treatment? It's a long and bumpy road.

The first surgeries for scoliosis were performed on French children by Jules Rene Guerin, a surgeon, in 1865 around the time when the American Civil War was coming to a close. Guerin devised a gruesome surgical technique that involved the severing of muscles and tendons. It didn't produce desirable outcomes, which should come as no surprise. In fact, these surgeries, which were incredibly performed on 1,349 child patients, led to one of the first instances of major medical dispute, prompting lawsuits from enraged family members (Ambrosio L., and Tanner, E; *Biomaterials for Spinal Surgery.* Amsterdam: Elsevier, 2012).

Many years later across the Atlantic, Dr. Russel Hibbs became the first person to perform a spinal-fusion surgery on a patient with scoliosis in 1914. Dr. Hibbs had been performing the surgery on other patients with different spinal deformities. It was so successful that he began to implement it to treat scoliosis caused by tuberculosis, a medical condition that was far more prevalent at the time. Hibbs's innovation caught on quickly among the medical establishment. It was quickly regarded as a groundbreaking treatment option for those with spinal deformities. It didn't take long for spinal-fusion surgery to become a widespread solution for a variety of spinal ailments, including scoliosis.

Less than thirty years after Dr. Hibbs's first spinal-fusion surgery for scoliosis, performing these operations on adolescents became quite common, usually to treat the effects of tuberculosis, which is known to cause problems with the spine. These surgeries led to numerous complications, largely because they utilized grafts from the patient's own shinbones in many cases. Doctors using this

177

procedure in the 1940s were able to achieve curve corrections of about 25 percent.

Later, Paul Harrington developed steel rods to aid in the surgical correction of scoliosis. Eventually, these rods were found to be ineffective unless they were combined with spinal-fusion surgical techniques. Still, patients lost all their flexibility in the areas of fusion. Recovery was grueling. And these surgeries could last for up to twelve hours. Patients were made to wear full-body casts after surgery, eventually transitioning into a brace that resembles today's Wilmington brace.

In the 1970s, surgical procedures for spinal fusion advanced yet again by including the usage of two Harrington rods. Not exactly a groundbreaking development, but it was enough to maintain spinal fusion as the standard for treatment of many spinal deformities.

One of the most recent developments in spinal-fusion surgery was the development of the pedicle screw, a new piece of hardware that allowed for the correction of scoliosis in different planes of space. The pedicle screw has allowed for decent rates of spinal correction, but it doesn't eliminate the possibility of complications.

This brings us to today. Very little has been done to improve or revolutionize spinal-fusion surgery for scoliosis in the last few decades. But it remains the standard model of treatment. It doesn't make sense, but when you consider the glacial pace of medical innovation, it becomes easier to understand why new, more effective methods of treatment have not caught on and become more popular.

Surgery is clearly no longer the gold standard for treating scoliosis, but that doesn't mean it should not exist. I believe surgery should remain as a last resort for patients who have tried other methods of treatment, but have not found success. Or it could be reserved for cases in which it is absolutely medically necessary. It certainly should not be performed with the frequency that is normal in today's standard model of treatment.

Really, there is no harm in treating the condition using non-surgical methods including scoliosis-specific chiropractic care. Alternative treatments like these aren't invasive. They don't create an irreversible new normal. They aren't terribly expensive, like surgery. Most importantly, these types of alternative treatments have been shown to reduce curvatures, restore function and allow patients to improve their quality of life considerably.

In cases where surgery is absolutely required, patients benefit from having gone through alternative methods of treatment. Scoliosis-specific chiropractic adjustments and exercises, for example, can build strength and flexibility in the spine, making it better able to withstand the rigors of surgery and recovery well. When patients come to the operating table having treated their spines with alternative methods, they are likely to experience far fewer complications as well.

The truth is that scoliosis surgery isn't inevitable. It should not be seen as the end goal of treatment. In fact, it should be avoided at all costs unless it becomes medically necessary as a last resort. Alternative methods of functional treatment, such as those used here at the Scoliosis Reduction Center, have been shown to provide patients with real, measurable results. With patients like you involved directly in scoliosis treatment, outcomes become more positive. With you in control of your own treatment, you get to decide for yourself what the gold standard really is. By treating your spine's condition with methods designed to restore function, you will become increasingly motivated by seeing results and feeling better over time. Clearly, this is the new gold standard for scoliosis treatment. Don't you agree?

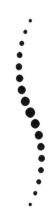

SECTION SIX

Effective Adult Scoliosis Treatment

WHAT DOES IT REALLY mean to treat your scoliosis effectively?

At this point in your life, the condition may not be progressing rapidly; it might actually be stabilized to a certain degree. But it's likely to be causing pain. And this pain grows every day, both in the number of locations of the body it affects as well as in its severity.

It is possible that pain is the factor that led to your discovery that you have scoliosis. Like many adults who have the condition, you've been able to put up with quite a bit in your grown-up life. But pain is a deal breaker, isn't it? Especially when it gets worse every single day. So now you have become serious about treating your scoliosis. You will do just about anything to experience a reduction in your pain levels.

Pain doesn't just hurt. It could be an indicator of further abnormal spinal progression over time. So you need to act in order to ensure that scoliosis doesn't become increasingly dominant in your life. Sadly, for adults who have scoliosis, the only options that

181

are typically recommended are pills to combat pain or surgery to "correct" the spine.

This isn't an ideal scenario, is it?

Thankfully, it's possible to reduce your pain and curvature at the same time through noninvasive treatments. In this section, you will learn all about the methods we use here at the Scoliosis Reduction Center, and why they tend to work so well for adult patients just like you.

CHAPTER TWENTY-ONE

Scoliosis-Specific Chiropractic: Why it Works

LET ME GUESS: YOU'RE here reading this book because you've done the research and concluded that traditional treatments aren't as promising as they are made out to be. They involve a lot of doing nothing on the way to expensive, invasive surgery. Knowing this, you have sought out alternative, more natural forms of treatment.

But you've probably found that although some modalities are more natural than undergoing surgery, they don't work in terms of providing relief for your scoliosis. Gym exercises, standard physical therapy techniques, and traditional chiropractic adjustments don't work. They might even cause more harm than good. They are severely limited because they focus on treating a patient's scoliosis symptoms rather than treating the scoliosis itself. What's more, these traditional treatments are usually performed to treat people who have suffered injuries. Therefore, treatments are completed slowly over a long period of time. This approach is wonderful for dealing with injuries, but it isn't effective for treating scoliosis, which in most cases is a developmental problem.

So what else is there? You are willing to commit to proactive, functional treatment, but finding the right modalities—and the right practitioners—is difficult. You want to do the hard work, but you're not about to waste time working hard on methods of treatment that only put you back at square one (or worse).

Scoliosis-focused chiropractic is a method you can trust because it's backed by real evidence of success. Rather than focusing on specific symptoms, scoliosis-focused chiropractic is used to treat the structural issues of your spine so you can reduce your curvature. This can lead to a dramatic reduction in pain. It's a systematic process that involves addressing the curvature directly, supporting and stabilizing the spine, and giving the patient the tools they need to sustain—and improve on—their results.

Have you heard the name Usain Bolt? As the world-record holder in the hundred-meter dash, he is considered to be the world's fastest human. He also has scoliosis, and has achieved all of his success while living with the condition. Surprising, isn't it? But it's not surprising to me and other scoliosis-focused chiropractors. Usain Bolt didn't opt for surgery, and thank goodness. Who knows if he would have achieved all his success if he had undergone surgery? Rather, he opted to undergo functional treatments for his scoliosis, with chiropractic at the center of it all.

You don't have to sacrifice your passions or the things in life that give you joy and meaning. In fact, by undergoing more functional treatments, you'll get more time and energy to pursue those things. You don't have to settle for surgery. With the help of a scoliosis-focused chiropractor, you can craft a treatment plan that reduces your curvature while bringing back your ability to live life to the fullest.

From My Perspective

My journey to becoming a scoliosis-focused chiropractor was spurred on by disillusionment with the traditional system. I was sick of all the watching and waiting patients were being told to endure. And I was tired of being unable to help them with traditional chiropractic methods. Thankfully, I discovered scoliosis-focused chiropractic, which has revolutionized my practice and brought real relief to countless patients just like you.

Under traditional treatment, spinal-fusion surgery is often recommended. To me, this is highly unnecessary. Patients should avoid surgery, if at all possible. They should not be funneled into it. And they certainly should not be given promises that surgery will make their pain go away or restore function to their lives.

Passive forms of treatment (i.e., watching and waiting on the way to surgery) are the standard for treating scoliosis these days, as they have been for decades. It all seems counterintuitive to me when there are alternative methods that have been shown to provide much more appealing results for patients.

In my view, successfully treating scoliosis means keeping some core principles in mind:

You Must Start with the Structure

In my view, it isn't possible to truly improve a patient's scoliosis without addressing the structural issues with their curvature first. In my practice at the Scoliosis Reduction Center, we begin our work at the heart of the issue and start functional treatment right away. We know that observation will only reveal further progression most likely. So we start by treating the patient immediately on a structural basis. There is no use in waiting.

Yes, you may have pain in your muscles and nerves. Your ability to function may be reduced by discomfort or pain in your joints as well. But treating your muscles, joints, and nerves fails to address the underlying structural realities of your spine. One way we can be sure the issue is structural is by performing movement analysis with X-rays. In these evaluations, we observe the curvature almost always retaining its shape and severity regardless of a patient's movements. If the issue were not structural, the curvature would shift in size and shape with the patient's movements.

You Must Begin Treatment as Soon as Possible

Early detection leads to better outcomes for scoliosis patients. So does early treatment. Continued progression only makes it more difficult to treat scoliosis, so it's important to begin treatment as quickly as possible. When we begin treatment early, it allows us to manipulate the spine and move it into the proper direction more easily. Restoring the greatest amount of function and mobility— while reducing pain and the effects of related symptoms—is our goal, so it makes no sense to wait to treat patients.

Reducing Curvatures Is Possible

If you think it isn't possible to reduce your abnormal curvature, you wouldn't even attempt it. That is, unfortunately, what the standard model of treatment tends to believe. I know that it is, in fact, possible to reduce abnormal curvatures by addressing the spine structurally. Scoliosis-specific chiropractic care can help move the spine into straighter alignment, and it's all done through natural means. There is no loss in strength or flexibility—these types of trade-offs are typical in surgical solutions, but not when we take a functional approach to treatment.

A Fully Comprehensive Treatment Plan

Under the traditional treatment model, the spine is stabilized with a rod. My goal is to strengthen and stabilize the spine through a functional approach so it can support itself. Making the spine stronger allows it to become more resistant to the progression of scoliosis. The approach I use is comprehensive. It involves multiple modes of treatment including scoliosis-specific chiropractic, active and passive rehabilitation, scoliosis-focused therapy, and corrective bracing.

A common problem arises when patients undergo this type of treatment: They must often go to multiple locations to receive the many different modes of treatment they need. This requires them to be in multiple places at different times, seeing numerous specialists for different aspects of their treatment. It is a lot to ask of any patient, and it typically serves to fragment the treatment approaches, making them less effective. My solution to this problem is putting all the different specialties under one roof. Here at the Scoliosis Reduction Center, my staff and I are trained in a wide range of treatments and modalities. Treatments can be combined in an additive fashion, which means they no longer work in competition with each other. We are better able to monitor patient progress this way too.

One of the reasons this approach is so effective is that we are able to concentrate and condense treatment. It's the inverse of the typical slow, injury-based approach, which is critical for reducing scoliosis. The duration of treatment is made as short as possible, but the intensity is increased. For some patents, the intensity level seems extreme, but it's done this way to ensure the greatest possible chance at reducing an abnormal spinal curvature. In my opinion, this level of intensity is necessary to combat the progression of scoliosis. Keep in mind that just because the treatment is intense doesn't mean that it's painful. In reality, you may exercise-like soreness initially, but it will reduce the amount of pain you feel that is related to your underlying structural condition.

After receiving treatment at the facility, patients aren't just sent home to rest and relax. They are given the go-ahead to go back home, but with a set of custom-designed treatment exercises that they can perform in order to sustain the progress they have made. This is one of the keys to this type of treatment's effectiveness, but it requires the patient to fully buy in to what we're doing. These exercises provide a huge benefit, though, because patients can perform them from the comfort of home, which helps them maintain the correction they've achieved.

Remember—traditional chiropractic produces, at best, mixed results for patients who have scoliosis. Even mild cases of scoliosis cannot be effectively treated using traditional chiropractic techniques. It is critical that if you see a chiropractor who has the specific training and expertise necessary to address your scoliosis.

Another major reason for the effectiveness of scoliosis-specific chiropractic is its combination with other important therapies like scoliosis-specific exercise and scoliosis-specific physical therapy. In order to be fully comprehensive, it's necessary to treat the structural issue of the spine from a number of directions.

Scoliosis-Specific Exercises

Scoliosis-specific exercises, which are sometimes referred to as *SSEs*, have been becoming popular around the globe in recent years after first arising in Europe. These exercises are designed to work in a corrective manner, and they are customized for each individual patient based on factors including curve type, curve size and the patient's physical abilities. They are also made up of various combinations of different movements, isometric exercises and exercises that work the body in a reflexive manner.

Among scoliosis-focused providers such as myself, an approach known as SEAS has emerged. This approach, which stands for *scientific exercise approach to scoliosis*, aims to improve the stability of the spine through active self-correction. The approach works by training neuromotor function in a way that stimulates a reflex to self-corrected posture during normal daily activities.

The exercises that you are prescribed by a scoliosis-focused provider will differ greatly from what you are accustomed to doing at the gym. These exercises are meant to influence attributes like your posture, coordination, and balance rather than build muscle mass. The exercises you're prescribed will also differ from those prescribed to other patients. It is necessary, in my opinion, to prescribe exercises on an individual basis because each patient's spine is different and responds differently to treatment. Furthermore, these exercises may seem strange at first because they don't always involve conscious contraction of the muscles. They are designed instead to train your neuromuscular function. This is yet another reason why customization is so crucial for success in your treatment.

Scoliosis-Specific Physical Therapy

Scoliosis-specific exercise is a lot different from regular, gym-based exercise. The same is true for scoliosis-specific physical therapy, which doesn't resemble most types of standard physical therapy.

The goal of this specialized type of physical therapy is to mobilize the spine into a corrected position in a passive manner. It uses multiple modes of treatment, including traction, de-rotation and vibration to achieve results. These types of treatments are usually performed using equipment designed specifically to address scoliosis.

An example of the type of equipment we use at the Scoliosis Reduction Center is the scoliosis traction chair. This piece of equipment is interesting because it works to reverse scoliosis by creating a mirror image of the patient's spine. This basic concept of creating a mirror image to treat scoliosis has been shown to be quite effective at reducing curvatures. Essentially, if a curvature goes to the right side of the body in a certain manner, this chair will create conditions where the spine is encouraged to curve in exactly the opposite direction. The result is usually a reduction in curvature, if not a restoration, in part, of the spine's normal curvature.

Other devices and techniques have been designed with this basic mirroring concept in mind. When used in combination with other modes of functional treatment, they can produce positive results for patients.

Corrective Bracing for Scoliosis

If you have ever imagined yourself in a traditional scoliosis brace, you might not be thrilled at the prospect of being prescribed a brace to treat your condition. Traditional braces are bulky, ugly and don't work to reduce abnormal spinal curvatures. Thankfully, big, bulky, hard-plastic braces that are common for adolescents are rarely, if ever, prescribed for adults.

Sometimes, adults are prescribed flexible braces for support and pain relief during exercise or other activities, but these aren't scoliosis braces. Furthermore, patients should understand that there is no chance of reducing a scoliosis with these types of braces.

Sometimes, adults can be treated effectively by a new brace design known as the ScoliBrace. This type of brace is designed to reduce scoliotic curvatures while wearing it rather than simply stabilizing the spine in a static position. Additionally, these braces are custom-designed for each patient using computer modeling software and advanced 3-D imaging. There are no one-size-fits-all options. They are more flexible, fitted, easier to wear and far more attractive than traditional braces as well.

In one notable case, a seventy-eight-year-old female patient experiencing pain, deformity, and reductions in function was prescribed a ScoliBrace to wear. Usage of the brace was, importantly, combined with a scoliosis-specific exercise regimen. Initially, this patient presented with significant coronal imbalance (when the upper spine becomes dislocated from the midline of the body) and a twenty-five-degree scoliosis curve to the right side in the lumbar region.

After fourteen months of treatment, the patient's pain was reduced noticeably. Their ability to function and enjoy a higher quality of life improved at the same time. Doctors also observed postural improvements in this patient. (*Source: https://www.scoli-care.com/adult-bracing-case-2/*)

Although it may not be reasonable to expect that a patient at the age of seventy-eight would be able to reduce their abnormal spinal curvature, anything is possible. At the very least, corrective bracing can help to restore healthier posture and reduce pain. All without undergoing surgery.

This fully comprehensive approach to treatment isn't normal, nor is it what most patients have come to expect from dealing with the traditional medical model. But it's the approach that has been shown to work the best for providing real, tangible results for adult scoliosis patients.

Scoliosis-specific chiropractic on its own would certainly be more helpful for patients than traditional chiropractic. And it's definitely more helpful than doing nothing. But it is as effective as it is because it is almost always combined with other noninvasive, functional therapies.

You may or may not be able to find relief through scoliosis-specific chiropractic and functional treatment, but the odds are in your favor. And don't you want to find out if it will work for you? If it doesn't, you can always return to the path that leads to surgery. If it *does* work, you will be saving yourself considerable time, energy, money, and enjoyment. There is nothing to lose.

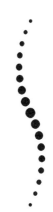

CHAPTER TWENTY-TWO

What Results Can You Expect from Treatment?

IF YOU'VE BEEN RESEARCHING scoliosis treatment options for adults, you have been treated to two main schools of thought. There is, of course, the well-established orthopedic model of treatment, which almost always leads patients toward surgery. This approach reacts to the underlying condition rather than treating it directly. It also focuses on treating symptoms during a period of observation leading up to surgery.

You've also found that there is an alternative approach that treats scoliosis in a functional, patient-centered manner. This is a proactive method of treating the condition that addresses the structural conditions of the patient's spine directly. It involves scoliosis-specific chiropractic care, in addition to other important therapies such as exercise, physical therapy, and corrective bracing, all of which are performed in a manner that is designed specifically to treat scoliosis.

This whole book has been about promoting the latter option, so I'm not trying to hide my agenda here—it should be obvious which side I'm on when it comes to the best way to treat adult patients like you. I have devoted my life and profession to treating scoliosis on a functional, structural level. The results my patients and I have achieved speak for themselves, and I'm happy to show my results, side by side, with those achieved by doctors using more traditional methods of treatment.

If you are wondering what you can expect from scoliosis treatment, I think it's useful to compare the two models against each other. Seeing how the two major models compare will allow you to make a sound decision regarding your treatment as you move forward. It may also reveal some facts that you were previously unaware of.

Let's take a look.

Scoliosis Diagnosis

Receiving a diagnosis marks the first step on your journey of treatment for the condition.

Traditional Treatment

Typically, adult patients begin experiencing pain or other symptoms that force them to seek medical attention and care. This usually leads them down roads where they treat their symptoms without treating the underlying causes. Patients tend to become disheartened and disillusioned with this cycle. They begin to suspect that their spines are the sources of their pain and discomfort. So they persist in seeking out solutions. Eventually, they may be diagnosed with scoliosis, either by a general practitioner or a provider who focuses on the condition specifically.

Often, adults with scoliosis have already been diagnosed with the condition in adolescence. But in their younger years, the condition was not painful, nor did it cause the problems they face in adulthood. So they failed to take action.

Chiropractic-Centered Treatment

Patients usually come to see me after becoming frustrated by providers in the traditional realm of treatment. They know something is going on with their spines and are seeking validation. Some of them suspect scoliosis because they were diagnosed with it in their youth. Others are pleased to know that they were right about the source of their condition all along. Actual diagnosis happens by examining multiple X-rays and scans of the body. To me, it's important to not just diagnose the condition, but to also determine its size, severity, and nature. That way, the patient and I can craft a custom treatment plan that's designed to work as quickly and effectively as possible to restore function, reduce pain and help the individual live their best life.

Treatment Goals for Adult Scoliosis Patients

What is the goal of treatment? You should not just assume that everyone wants to reduce your curvature and restore your function.

Traditional Treatment

The goal of treatment under the traditional model isn't always clear. Is the goal to avoid surgery or to prepare you for eventual surgery? Is the goal to make your life better or to have you sit and wait until you become a viable candidate for an operation? In many cases, the goal of treatment under the traditional model is to avoid doing anything at all. That is probably not good enough for you, is it?

Chiropractic-Centered Treatment

Here at the Scoliosis Reduction Center, our goal for each patient, regardless of age, ability, or severity, is to reduce their abnormal spinal curvature as much as possible. Reducing the curvature is the key to reducing pain, restoring function, and helping the patient live the life they want to live. We are looking for real, measurable results, and we are usually able to achieve them with adult patients.

Observing the Condition

Observation is often used in place of action when it comes to traditional treatments. Is observation useful in alternative treatment as well?

Traditional Treatment

Upon diagnosis of scoliosis, the patient will be directed to watch and wait rather than go into treatment for the condition. Observation is recommended instead of action. For adult patients, doctors want to see if the curve will progress to the point at which it requires surgery. Until that point, they will treat the patient's symptoms rather than treating the structural issues at the heart of the condition.

Chiropractic-Centered Treatment

My preferred approach doesn't involve watching and waiting. I see no value in it, to be honest. In my opinion, a diagnosis should be seen as an opportunity to take action. Watching and waiting will only reveal further progression. By getting to work on treatment as soon as possible, patients and I are able to increase the chances of causing a reduction in curvature and relief from the symptoms they are experiencing. Observation is useful, but only to check on the results we are working to achieve with our actions.

Bracing for Scoliosis

It's common to use bracing to treat scoliosis. However, there are significant differences between the bracing techniques used under the traditional treatment model versus those used by scoliosis-specific providers like me.

Traditional Treatment

Under the traditional treatment model, adolescents are considered candidates for bracing with devices like the Boston brace or Milwaukee brace. These devices are hard, rigid, and unforgiving. They don't work to reduce abnormal spinal curvatures, either. Rather, they squeeze the spine in an effort to stop progression. This is actually not as helpful as bracing that pushes the spine into the corrected position, but doctors continue to prescribe traditional braces for younger patients.

For adults, traditional braces are rarely recommended. There is too much that can go wrong in terms of the body's degeneration if an adult were to wear a traditional brace for extended periods of time. So this treatment option is effectively removed from the table when it comes to treating adult scoliosis with traditional medical methods.

Chiropractic-Centered Treatment

As described in the previous chapter, bracing is a useful method for treating adults who have scoliosis. However, the bracing technology that we use is more corrective. Plus, it's designed specifically for each patient. It pushes the spine into a corrected position rather than squeezing it, which can be harmful. This type of bracing, crucially, is combined with strengthening exercises and it's designed to address the condition of scoliosis in a three-dimensional manner, which is necessary in order to achieve results from treatment. The brace we use is a specific invention known as the ScoliBrace, and it's appropriate for patients at any age, depending on their specific situation.

Exercises for Scoliosis

Physical fitness is very useful in treating scoliosis because fit bodies tend to respond to treatment better. But is it possible to use specific exercises in combination with other therapies that aid treatment?

Traditional Treatment

Doctors who treat scoliosis under the traditional model usually don't recommend exercise to patients, even though such exercises might strengthen the spine and its surrounding muscles. In fact, they might even discourage adult patients like you from participating in exercise or physical fitness routines. Patients are usually told to take it easy so they don't damage their bodies as they watch and wait.

Chiropractic-Centered Treatment

Exercise and physical fitness are cornerstones of health, which is why they should be incorporated into treatment for adult scoliosis in most cases. Scoliosis-specific exercises help patients in a number of ways: They build strength, improve flexibility, and work alongside other therapies to reduce abnormal curvatures. These exercises aren't like traditional gym exercises. They differ in that they are designed to make the body more limber and flexible, not to build muscle mass. When adults engage in these types of exercises while maintaining a baseline level of fitness, it can improve their odds of scoliosis-focused treatment success considerably.

Physical Therapy for Scoliosis

Physical therapy is a treatment modality that is used to address a number of injuries and conditions. Though it's often difficult to endure, it is key to a patient's ability to build strength, function and stamina.

Traditional Treatment

Physical therapy is rarely recommended for adult scoliosis patients under the traditional model. Remember, the standard approach involves watching and waiting, so taking action with physical therapy would run counter to the values of this model. What happens is patients usually end up doing nothing when they could be engaged in therapies that help them achieve their goals.

Chiropractic-Centered Treatment

Scoliosis-specific physical therapy, which is different from standard physical therapy, is one of the fundamental components of treatment under the functional model. When combined with scoliosis-specific chiropractic, exercise, and (sometimes) corrective bracing, it can help adult patients gain strength and mobility much more quickly. As described in the previous chapter, we use specialized devices such as the scoliosis traction chair to help patients reduce their curvatures.

It's important to keep in mind that if you plan to treat your scoliosis using physical therapy, you should seek scoliosis-specific physical therapy providers. Otherwise, you could fail to get the results you want or even set your treatment back.

Surgery for Scoliosis

Ask the average person what can be done to treat scoliosis, and they will probably reply with, "Surgery." But is surgery really the best option for people who have this condition in adulthood?

Traditional Treatment

Expensive, invasive, and potentially risky surgery represents the end goal of the conventional treatment model. If you're getting treated under the medical model, you will probably be recommended for surgery at some point if your curve continues to progress. And as we know, curves always progress to some degree. All the watching and waiting you do only serves to ensure the continued progression. X-rays are taken. You will be examined. You will experience much more pain in your body. Eventually, surgery will become necessary.

Once a patient has surgery, a new story begins. And it isn't necessarily a better one.

Chiropractic-Centered Treatment

There is no surgical solution under the chiropractic-centered model for scoliosis treatment. Surgery is the one thing we are trying to avoid. If you are attracted to the chiropractic-centered model, you need to know that it will steer you away from surgery and toward solutions that strive to correct your spine's abnormal curvature through more natural means.

Even though the average patient in my practice is above the surgical threshold, my goal is always to help patients avoid surgery. It should only be a last resort for those who have tried all other options unsuccessfully. This is the most dramatic difference between the treatment approach I believe in and the one the medical establishment has been promoting for decades. To me, the functional, patient-centered approach is incredibly helpful even when patients don't respond to it. Some patients will ultimately require surgery. But the treatments almost always improve a patient's overall health, and prepare them for a better surgical outcome.

Can You Tell the Difference?

Two potential paths of treatment. Two different sets of results.

At this point in your life, do you really have the time to watch and wait while your condition continues to worsen? Do you have the ability to endure ever-increasing amounts of pain and discomfort? I don't think so.

There are real differences between these two approaches, and it is clear to me that one is a lot more effective than the other—the functional, scoliosis-focused approach centered on scoliosis-specific chiropractic care. However, the traditional model has history, popularity, and the status quo on its side. Thankfully, now that you're armed with the facts about these two differing treatment paths, you can make the decision that is perfect for you and your specific situation.

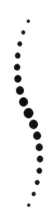

CHAPTER TWENTY-THREE

You Have Control

I BET YOU ARE quite accustomed to feeling like you're not the one in control of your life. It's a very unpleasant feeling, especially if you have raised children, advanced in your career, and done everything right in your life. The fact is that if you're an adult with scoliosis, you're probably living in pain and discomfort much of the time. That makes it incredibly difficult to take on each day with a positive attitude. It makes it hard to hold the belief that you can take your life into your own hands and improve it.

The fact is that you have control over your life. You have choices available to you. There are options in terms of how you move forward with your condition. You can even look forward to having fun with your life, which might be something you thought was off the table. It's true: adults with scoliosis can see improvements. Not only in the measurable curvatures of their spines, but also in the way they feel and go about living life.

You don't have to consider yourself a victim of your condition. You can, in fact, take control and be in charge of what happens next. The possibilities that have been placed in front of you up until now may not have been very attractive. But now there is a chance for you to live the rest of your life the way you want. On your terms. Without the excruciating pain or limitations you've come to know so well from your scoliosis.

Some Tips for Showing Off Your Style with Scoliosis

I love it when my patients start regaining their confidence.

For many adult patients, I can tell their confidence has returned when they start paying attention to their sense of style once again. They began their journeys feeling a little low, with very little regard to things like fashion. It's hard to care about looking good when you're in pain. But over time, I see patients feel less pain and gain increasing amounts of self-esteem. They begin to look at themselves in the mirror again, seeing themselves in a whole new way.

You may be wondering if you will ever get your sense of fun or fashion back. Well, I can tell you that it is possible. In fact, it's something that you should look forward to as you begin your own personal journey of treatment.

Scoliosis brings a higher degree of difficulty, though, when it comes to picking out the right clothes and wearing them in a way that's flattering to your body.

The visible symptoms of scoliosis cause clothes to become ill-fitting or uncomfortable to wear. And the more visible symptoms you have, the more difficult it will be for you to build a wardrobe that expresses who you are fashionably. This can turn into a challenge that presents itself every single day.

One tip is to avoid clothes that fit too tightly. When you wear clothes that fit too snugly to your body, it makes the asymmetry more easily recognizable. Over the course of day, this can be very uncomfortable as well.

Some items to consider adding to your wardrobe include looser options such as hoodies, shawls, blazers, cardigans, and jackets. Layering these items with T-shirts and other garments is also a great way to show off your fashion while remaining comfortable with how you feel and appear to the world.

If you have a high hip, which is common for people with scoliosis, you can accessorize with a wider bag. This can make you appear more balanced. Be careful when selecting a bag, though; you want to make sure it isn't too heavy or is capable of causing pain.

Sometimes, the length of pants is an issue. One leg fits great, but the other is too short or too long. My advice is to purchase pants that fit well on your longer leg. Then you can hem the other side appropriately. This is something that is easily done by most tailors, but you can probably learn how to do it yourself with a little YouTube research.

Dresses and skirts might also appear to be uneven. This is remedied by pinning the hem of the garment to appear straight while you're wearing it. Then, it is possible to stitch a new hem that causes the garment to look perfect as you wear it. It won't look straight on the hanger, but that's okay.

As your confidence continues to grow, you will notice that more and more clothes seem to look and fit good on you. That's because confidence is the key to a great appearance. And as long as you continue your recommended functional treatments, your confidence is likely to continue growing.

In my opinion, noninvasive, conservative treatment of scoliosis is the only approach that makes sense. It's a highly individualized condition, with no two cases that are alike. Every spine tells its own story at its own pace. That being the case, why would anyone ever move forward with a one-size-fits-all treatment approach? To me, it is absolutely necessary to address the condition on a case-by-case basis. And it's vital to ensure that the patient feels in control of what is happening to them. Treatment plans will involve similar strategies, but each patient gets their own path forward, based on the way the condition has manifested in them individually and what their specific goals are.

Most importantly, I take time to talk to my patients so I can understand what they want to get out of their treatment. Patients aren't used to this. You are also not used to it, are you?

But what if you really could take matters in your own hands? The results could be pretty amazing. You should be the one at the center of your treatment. That is the only way you will achieve your vision of success. First, you have to spend time figuring out what you want and what you're willing to do to achieve it. Then, it's necessary to make sure your vision aligns with those who can help you get to where you are going on your scoliosis journey.

Now that you know the realities of the treatment options that have been presented to you, it's possible to make informed decisions that don't feel like a shot in the dark. You really do have all the control you need over your life. Will you use it to act?

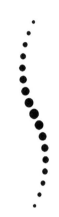

CHAPTER TWENTY-FOUR

It's Not Too Late; Now Is the Time to Act

EARLY DETECTION AND EARLY treatment are important when it comes to treating scoliosis effectively. Taking action as soon as possible is truly the best way to confront the condition. Yet here you are as an adult with scoliosis. It's possible that you have been living with it since adolescence. It's possible that it developed in adulthood. But you've not taken action up until this point, so you might be feeling guilty.

The truth is that it isn't too late for you to act. And action doesn't have to mean signing up for surgery, contrary to popular belief. You can pursue functional-treatment options now that could have a profound effect on how you live the rest of your life.

Although you have not taken action yet, doing so now is much better than waiting another ten, twenty years or more to finally seek help.

I would also argue that you've already taken action, even if you don't know it.

The fact that you picked up this book means, to me, that you aren't convinced that the traditional model of treating scoliosis really works. You're skeptical of what you've been told by "experts." You have a sense that something is going on with your spine, and I hope you've received validation here. If you have already been diagnosed with scoliosis, I hope that taking action by reading this book has opened your eyes to what is possible.

You don't have to live in fear. You don't have to live with hopelessness or uncertainty. You can actually work to reduce the excruciating levels of pain you might be experiencing. It is all possible if you act now.

Basically, you have a couple of choices available to you right now as an adult with scoliosis:

One is to do nothing or continue observation of the condition. In other words, this is watching and waiting. This option ensures that you will continue to endure pain and discomfort. It keeps you busy fighting symptoms while your structural condition continues its progression in your body. This option is no good.

The other option is the obvious one to take, in my opinion. It's the one that puts you in the center of your own treatment. It is the option that uses a custom treatment plan designed just for you and your spine. It's the option that keeps you from having to undergo surgery unless it becomes absolutely necessary. It is the option that can relieve your pain from the source and restore function to your life. It's the option that can extend the quality of your life and add years of enjoyment to your existence.

Now that you have come this far, I can't imagine that you would want to pursue option number one. So the choice for you should be quite clear. Scoliosis-focused treatment that is guided by a scoliosis specialist is the way to go if you are an adult who has the condition. It helps you avoid pain and avoid surgery. And I can guide you through your recovery.

What will you do now? The choice is yours to make.

I appreciate you taking the time to read this book. I believe that with your newfound knowledge, you're equipped to make the best possible choices to treat your adult scoliosis. You can also be part of a new movement in understanding scoliosis—one that spreads the word about functional treatment. I hope you are inspired.

To learn more, contact the Scoliosis Reduction Center, located in gorgeous Celebration, Florida, today. Our doors are open, and we would love to see you walk through them. Call us at 321-939-2328 to talk to one of our amazing staff members, and be sure to check out all the great information on our website at scoliosisreductioncenter.com.

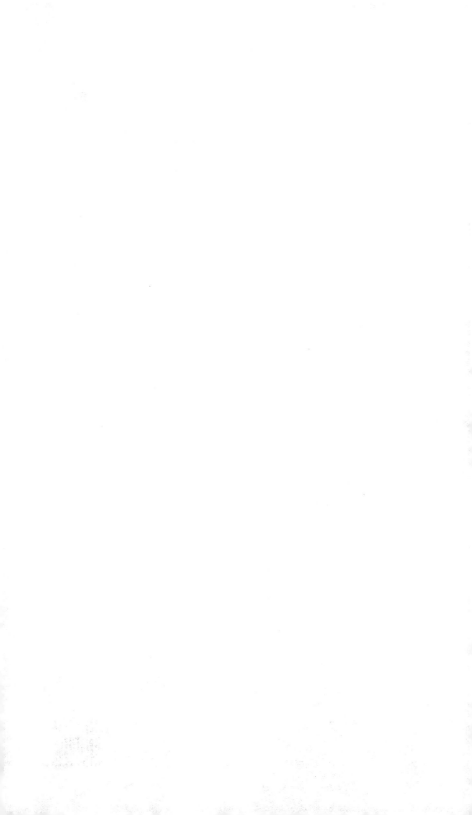

CPSIA information can be obtained
at www.ICGtesting.com
Printed in the USA
BVHW051749260323
661168BV00012B/346